Curriculum Design and Development

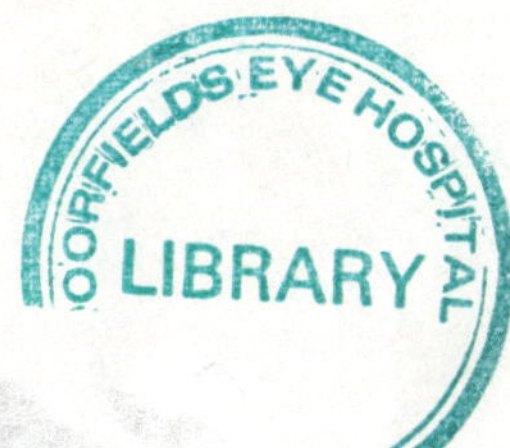

Curriculum Design and Development

A practical manual for nurse educators

T.W. BURRELL MA, Ph.D
Royal Shrewsbury Hospital School of Nursing

IN ASSOCIATION WITH

SHEILA M. ASTBURY, SRN, RSCN, RNT
Director of Nurse Education

PETER M. MACKAY, SRN, RMN, RCNT, DN(Lond).
Senior Tutor, Post-Basic Studies

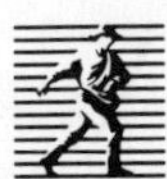

Prentice Hall

New York London Toronto Sydney Tokyo

First published 1988 by
Prentice Hall International (UK) Ltd,
66 Wood Lane End, Hemel Hempstead,
Hertfordshire, HP2 4RG
A division of
Simon & Schuster International Group

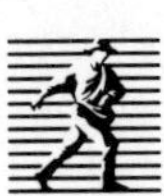

Printed and bound in Great Britain by
A. Wheaton & Co Ltd, Exeter.

British Library Cataloguing in Publication Data

Burrell, T.W. (Tom W.) *1923 –*
    Curriculum design and development: a
    practical manual for nurse educators.
    1. Great Britain. Nurses. Professional
    education. Curriculum. Planning
    I. Title   II. Astbury, Sheila M.
    III. MacKay, Peter M.
    610.73'07'1141

    ISBN 0-13-195611-6

---

1 2 3 4 5 92 91 90 89 88

ISBN 0-13-195611-6

Contents

Preface

With the publication and widespread discussion of the draft and final proposals of *Project 2000*, nursing in the United Kingdom has embarked upon a phase of development that is likely to lead to the adoption of new and extended aims, new methods of operation and more rigorous standards for professional work. There is a strong case for regarding the curricula of our schools and departments of nursing as a key factor in these developments and we have been directed to reappraise and reshape them.

New generations of nurses must be introduced to new or revitalised knowledge, attitudes and skills, or confirmed afresh in those which will remain indispensable in something like their present form, in the design of these local curricula.

Thereafter, constant review and modification, the essentials of curriculum development, should ensure that nursing will always be kept relevant to the changing demands and opportunities of succeeding decades through the basic and continuing education of nurses.

The purpose of this manual is to reassure nurse educators that there *is* a systematic, if somewhat lengthy, procedure available for curriculum design and development and to provide a relatively brief and simple step-by-step guide to the stages involved, together with an extended commentary on each step.

The procedure recommended here is not, however, so brief and simple that it lacks the necessary depth and rigour of treatment required by an essentially academic task, and a serious attempt has been made to avoid 'jargon' without losing precision in thought and language.

Perhaps it would be useful at this point to indicate the exact scope of this book. It is *not* intended to serve as an authoritative treatise on the philosophy of nursing or the theory of education; it has *no* startlingly fresh revelations to offer in the matters of nursing models or the nursing process although these are all important ingredients in forming a curriculum. It is *not* intended to debate the pros and cons of the various approaches to curriculum design and development because each of these approaches is essentially a special view-point which emerges from the corporate attitudes and spirit of the teaching staff and students in each particular school or department. This is reflected in the way in which they apply their corporate thinking to the creation of an individual, possibly unique, atmosphere or set of values in which to conduct the everyday tasks of teaching and learning and living in their own hospital or college community: it cannot and should not be prescribed by an outsider and this text is not intended to be prescriptive in that way.

On the other hand, other systems or models of curriculum design are available but they are usually intended for spheres other than the professional services such as nursing; for example, they may be prepared for use in primary schools or in industrial apprenticeship regimes. Of course, there is no reason why you should not explore these systems and models and their associated theories once you have mastered this procedure. If you wish to satisfy yourself that what you have done or propose to do will stand the usual tests of academic rigour across a broader spectrum of experience, you will find a short reading list at the end of this book to help you.

By this process of elimination you should now have concluded that the present purpose is to provide a detailed guide to the construction and maintenance of the basic curriculum structure, somewhat in the manner of a procedure manual, having always in view the aim of educating learner nurses to perform their difficult, expanding and rather imprecise role with the greatest possible professional efficacy, distinction and joy.

Although reference is made throughout this book to nurses and to education for nursing, the text should be equally suitable for the needs of curriculum design and development teams in other parts of the health services, for example, in the midwifery and paramedical sectors, in all parts of the world where health care services are in the process of being established, remodelled or updated. However, it is to nurses of all grades that this book is respectfully and affectionately dedicated, in particular those chiefly concerned in its production, Sheila M. Astbury and Peter Mackay, since the writer has shared their world and valued their companionship for several happy years. Above all, my thanks are due to my wife, Evelyn, who has been my dearest and most constructive critic for many happy years and has contributed Step 5.

A serious attempt has been made to ensure that this book remains, as its sub-title implies, a very practical manual on how to design, construct and test a curriculum for a school or department of nursing. The writers have sought to avoid lengthy investigations of purely theoretical interest to educationists and to avoid wasting the time of very busy nurses and nurse-teachers with material which is not of immediate and practical concern to them as curriculum designers and developers. Our aim has been explanation without obfuscation.

It must be clear that the book is directed primarily towards the sector of general nursing and that correspondingly less attention has been directed towards the particular problems of, say, psychiatric nursing or post-basic education. Yet it is hoped that everybody concerned in health service education and training and, indeed, those working in other fields altogether, may find something to help them in their work.

Good fortune, and good evaluation results!

Please note that in the interests of clarity the nurse is categorised as 'she' and the client as 'he'.

The general expression 'client' is generally preferred to 'patient', 'health-care consumer' or any of the other terms now available in growing numbers. In spite of its somewhat commercial image, it reflects professional usage.

Chapter 1

Some essential preliminaries

What is a curriculum?

A brief, but adequate, definition is that a curriculum is the whole set of influences and events, both planned and unforeseen, which impinge upon students during their period of education and which will, sooner or later, affect their ability to understand and achieve the aims of the course and, indeed, of the wider arena for which they are being educated. The more systematic the planning of the curriculum the more effective the course of education will be in helping them to achieve their aims.

Why have a curriculum?

At this early stage, perhaps before you are wholly committed to curriculum design or development, you are entitled to know the reasons for having a curriculum as opposed to not having one at all. This latter stance may be defended more readily than one might imagine since, given an open-ended learning situation, that is, one with no pre-conditions or external constraints and blessed with unlimited resources, a very effective way to proceed might well be to allow the students to explore the workings of local health services, explore the literature, examine particular issues in depth with those already working in the services and discuss the apparent implications of all that they encounter. They might turn to their tutors only for clarification of obscure issues and puzzling practices. In this way, over a long period of time and without any formal curriculum, those students who had shown their dedication by staying the course would probably have arrived at a comprehensive, realistic and possibly highly critical understanding of the systems which they had discovered and might have acquired a formidable range of relevant skills and commendable attitudes, leavened with a healthy cynicism. They might, in due course, generate a brisk wind of change throughout the profession and the health services by their aptitude for research and their willingness to innovate.

On the other hand, the situation is *not* open-ended, if only because in the first place the profession is now required by edict to review and revise its curricula. Fortunately, from most points of view, this is permitted to be done as a local exercise within each school or department rather than being imposed by a central 'think-tank': thus we are all able to contribute from a much wider pool of wisdom and experience than would otherwise be the case and also tailor our curricula to local needs and opportunities.

Time and resources are not only finite but in short supply and the whole process is subject to cost-benefit analysis and, indeed, many other layers of external constraint. Statutory requirements are placed upon members of the profession. The United Kingdom Central Council for Nursing, Midwifery and Health Visiting (UKCC) has requirements regarding the Code of Professional Conduct, with its views on the nurse's accountability to the patients, the profession and the public; cooperation with colleagues; confidentiality of information; qualms of conscience; and the duty of undertaking self-development and facilitating similar efforts by others. Through its Training Rules (Nurses, Midwives and Health Visitors Rules Approval Order 1983, No. 873) Appendix B, paragraph 18(1), the UKCC specifies that courses shall provide opportunities to 'enable the student to accept responsibility for her personal professional development' and to acquire the competencies required to operate in nine specified functional areas 'related to the care of the particular type of patient with whom she is likely to come in contact when registered'. Only a formal curriculum can accommodate such constraints.

Further, the English National Board for Nursing, Midwifery and Health Visiting (ENB) is typical of many boards in retaining the right to grant or withhold approval of a course or curriculum. The ENB requires the submission by the school of an application which must specify in detail, under a considerable array of headings and sub-headings, all relevant information about the school. This includes its policies, staff, accommodation, resources and facilities and, as regards the proposed curriculum, its date of commencement, membership, finances, management, content, structure, assessment methods and so on. This information must be submitted at least a year before the proposed date of commencement and is followed by a Board inspection of the institution concerned. It is clear that such examining and certificating boards would almost certainly have a supervisory role such as that outlined even if the schools were to acquire a greater degree of autonomy than they have at present. This degree of supervision is not unreasonable but demands curriculum design skills of a high order if broader educational issues are not to be obscured.

There are also the expectations of the service sector to be anticipated, and the expectations of the students themselves are of considerable interest and importance Their approach to their education involves the gradual development of acute observation, reporting and analysis of findings, while the synthesis or constructing of a better system, policy or procedure from the fragments of the old one, even on paper, demands a high degree of imagination and practical planning. These are high-level intellectual skills which can be expected to emerge only towards the end of a carefully organised course of higher education. They are a product of the educational process, embodied in a carefully prepared curriculum, rather than tools to be brought by the students, ready-honed, at the beginning of the course. It is also fair to say that students in a new and unfamiliar vocational field normally expect and welcome the guidance and discipline of a well-organised and publicised curriculum and should not be denied the support which it offers. The duties of nursing are likely to be regarded by the students as being of such importance and gravity that they may be unwilling to risk the omission of any element that might contribute to their own future competence and, ultimately, to the patients' welfare.

The justification for the design of a curriculum in education for nursing lies in the undoubted fact that it is the best guarantee that all these criteria will be foreseen and incorporated in the proposed course for the benefit of all concerned.

Who should design and develop the curriculum?

The work is onerous and, in addition to the imaginative interpretation of the nursing needs of the next two decades and the exercise of logical thinking, involves the painstaking manipulation of masses of details. It is a task, therefore, for a closely integrated and mutually supportive team which should not only complete the curriculum design but should also be kept in being for the less exciting but equally vital function of reviewing, revising and revalidating the curriculum over a period of many years. Updated it must be; perfected it will never be!

The 'perfect' curriculum for any one institution is probably unattainable and no tears should be spilled over that. The search for perfection can so easily relapse into stagnation and a workable curriculum is essentially dynamic in the true sense of that much over-used word. Thus, the curriculum will almost certainly remain in a constant cycle of change as the members of the development team strive to keep it relevant to changing conditions, new opportunities for growth and new challenges to those being educated under its aegis. It is pointless, therefore, to expend unlimited hours of thought in the attempt to 'get it right first time'. This is almost sure to founder in boredom, if not actual conflict between members of the team, before the first step is completed. It is sufficient to achieve a reasonable and agreed approach to the problem as it is seen locally. Once this agreed foundation is established a useful curriculum can be designed. Subsequent cycles of development carried out on the same lines and in the same spirit will ensure that stagnation is kept at bay and maximum relevance to current conditions is maintained.

In order to avoid the almost inevitable accusations of living in an ivory tower, remote from the service needs of the parent institution and from the suffering of students, the team should be representative of all the staff and student hierarchies in the nursing, medical and paramedical sectors as well as including selected members of the teaching staff of the school concerned and such specialists as post-basic tutors, librarians and allocation officers. It is reasonable to enlist the services of an academic consultant in curriculum design if this would serve to integrate and speed up the work of the team, but no consultant should be allowed near the nursing content of the curriculum without strict supervision since experts can wreak havoc when they operate independently in a speciality other than their own. Perhaps an acceptable manual would be a useful safeguard against both excesses and over-timidity in the team's approach to its task.

Probably ten is an optimum number of members for the team in most circumstances since this number is small enough to permit members to confer effectively in committee and to acquire mutual empathy, but large enough to be split up occasionally into specialised sub-groups with delegated responsibilities and also to maintain the momentum of the work through the inevitable absences of members on other duties or because of illness. In an ideal world members would be relieved of all other duties for the duration of the design process, probably for over a year of full-time work on the project.

It is vital that all members should be able to contribute elements such as imaginative creativity, cooperation and good humour and, above all perhaps, the ability to work in a dedicated and concentrated manner and to make decisions with firmness while maintaining a consistently high rate of output. Variety of membership also facilitates one of the most important requirements of the process: the maintenance of a constant flow of information in both directions between the curriculum team and their constituency in the service divisions and the students' organisation. Decisions must appear never to be imposed upon the profession.

A final word before you take the plunge

There is no magic formula for this work: there are no short cuts in the process of curriculum design and development and there is no 'off-the-peg' assistance in your struggle to construct local solutions to your education and training problems or in your determination to provide a better and constantly improving service to patients in the face of what might appear at the moment a bleak future for us all. It is important that you contribute to this curriculum process, in addition to the above attributes, a burning desire to do everything you can to ensure that your younger colleagues achieve their maximum potential without undue stress. If you didn't have this attribute already you would probably not be where you are; it is only a question of redirecting it into this new and most worthwhile undertaking.

If you find that this book, like some others on curriculum design and development, appears to adopt a rather 'idealistic' approach to nursing, please remember that this is the only opportunity that you will ever have to start from the standpoint of what *should* be, rather than from the stark reality of what *is*. Curriculum design is all about ideals.

Chapter 2

How to design a curriculum: a brief step-by-step outline

Taking the plunge!

In this chapter you will find an outline of the procedure for designing a curriculum for a school or department of nursing. You should begin by having a close look at the summary diagrams (Figures 2.1 and 2.2) before reading this chapter. Once you have read and absorbed the contents you should be able to write down on one side of a sheet of A4 paper a list of the necessary steps in the procedure, in the right order, together with a few words explaining the purpose and nature of each step. You might then move on to the remaining sections of the book and read about each step in greater depth and consider the examples which they offer, particularly as regards the method of carrying out each part of the procedure quickly and smoothly and then using its product as the basis for activity in the next step in the logical process. In this way you should master the procedure stage by stage and carry your knowledge and skill forward to a successful conclusion.

STEP 1   Defining the nature of nursing: a 'philosophy'

Given that you are prepared to accept the necessity for a new curriculum for the reasons offered in the previous section, or others similar to them, it would follow that it is of the utmost importance to define very carefully the nature of the vocation for which your students are to be prepared. This is not a waste of time, a mere exercise in an academic vacuum, because upon your answer will depend the whole nature of your curriculum and the nature of the impact upon the profession by your output of qualified nurses. In effect you will be shaping the future for better or for worse in your own locality and perhaps much further afield.

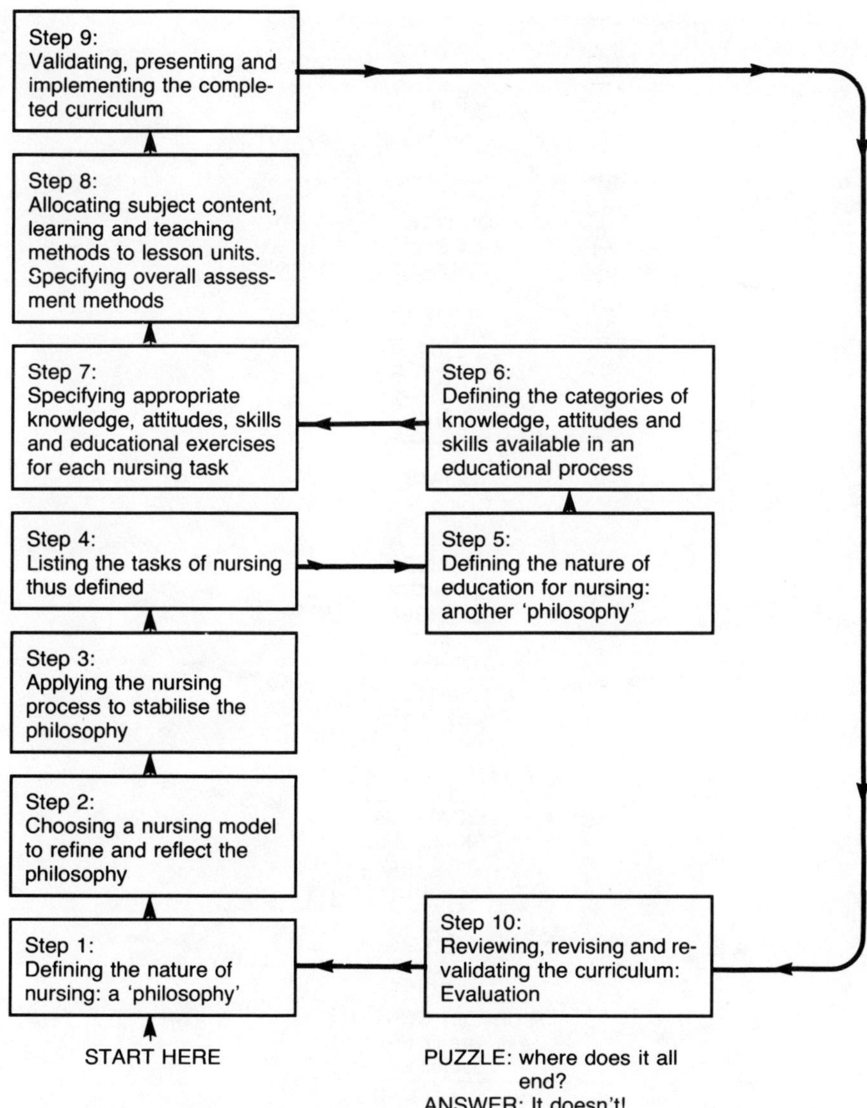

The cycle of curriculum design and development, as shown here, is a recognised procedure that ensures the work is done thoroughly and logically and that no important steps are left out. It is not difficult; only infinitely time-consuming. It is not frustrating; only infinitely intriguing and satisfying.

Figure 2.1 A flow-chart of curriculum design.

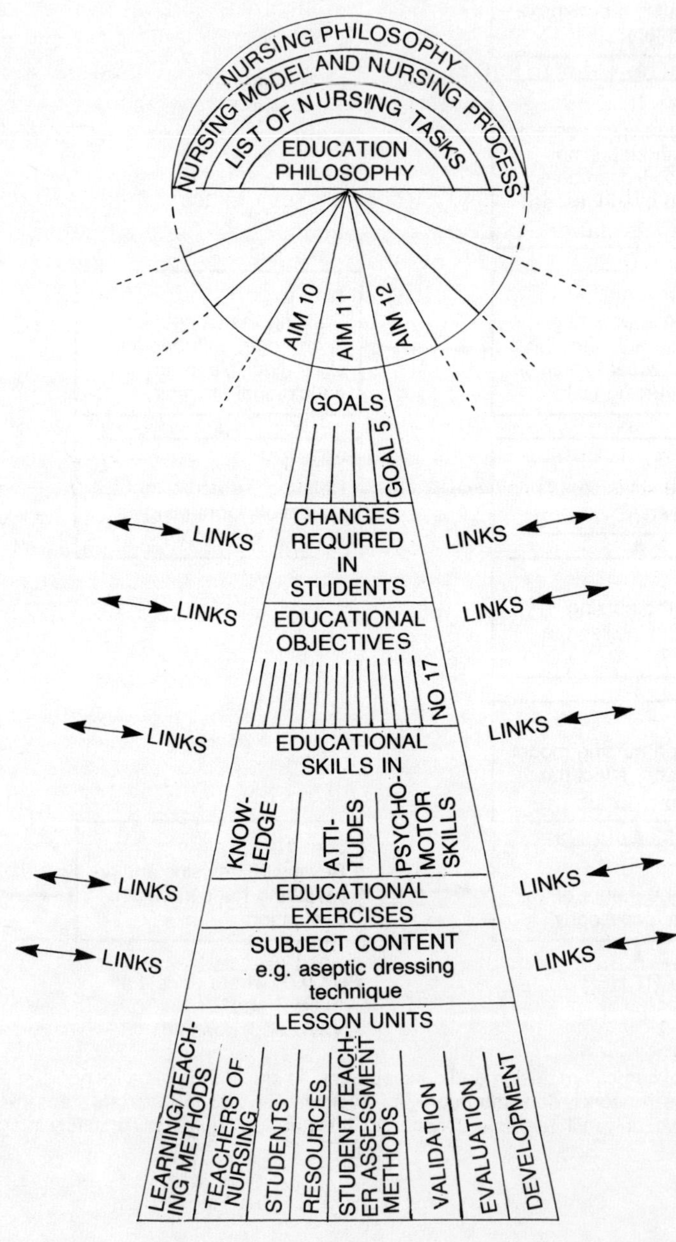

Figure 2.2   Curriculum design and development: a conspectus.

What is required, then, is a philosophy of nursing to underpin all your planning. This is inescapable and cannot be allowed to discourage the curriculum design team. There is an obligatory element in that Statutory, UKCC, ENB and Health Authority requirements must be accommodated, but restrictions due to limited institutional facilities, funding and staffing can and should be ignored at this stage because one is striving to express an ideal, unsullied by such mundane considerations which might, of course, be removed or overcome at a later stage.

The fact that no-one has yet been clever or lucky enough to produce a universally acclaimed philosophy of nursing should not deter you. The team should be broadly based, as already suggested, and sufficiently well-intentioned and amicable to arrive at an agreed statement which reflects an adequate degree of local consensus on the outline of such a philosophy which will serve as a basis for the work to follow.

In addition to the constraints mentioned above, there should be positive elements reflecting an attitude towards the patients and some acknowledgement of what a nurse should know and do, but, above all perhaps, some statement as to what kind of person a nurse should *be*. The purpose of this process is to produce a person who shall be so completely immersed in nursing that he or she instinctively thinks and acts as a nurse in any conceivable situation in which it is appropriate to do so. The local statement of the philosophy of nursing must be so comprehensive, within the span of three or four paragraphs, that from it alone can be drawn the fine threads of expressed and implied requirements which, when woven into a curriculum and implemented in practice, will produce this kind of specialised personality.

If you feel inclined to argue against this on the grounds that it amounts to indoctrination of the student, one can only agree wholeheartedly. In the hands of a benign and democratically accountable authority it can be used to expose and promote wholly admirable resources within those who voluntarily cooperate with it after a full and frank briefing. If they do not like the situation, students can always withdraw from the course or stay with it and seek to have their grievances investigated and redressed.

You have here an opportunity to rethink the whole purpose and nature of nursing. You may, in fact, emerge with a vision which coincides almost exactly with what you have been thinking and doing in your work for many years past, but the chances are that you will emerge with something significantly different and promising a better service to your patients. In any case, as nurse educators, you will have thought this through for yourselves and will now be aware of the necessity, and the methods, of establishing a vision and using it as a signpost to the future; a future which you can play a large part in shaping.

Baroness Warnock has said (*The Times*, Profile, 21 March, 1985) that every true profession should have 'a central and shared idea which makes the profession one'. This central and shared idea, placed in its locally negotiated setting, is crucial to your process of curriculum design and development.

STEP 2   Choosing a nursing model to refine and reflect the philosophy of nursing

A nursing model is simply an organised set of ideas which displays, in words or diagrams, the essential features of a proposed activity, reduced to its essence. Your choice of a nursing model expresses whatever particular view of the nature and purposes of nursing was specified in, or could be inferred from, your philosophy of nursing. It imparts purpose and direction to the philosophy and gives it wings.

Any one of the better known models: Roy, Riehl, Rogers, Roper and the others, may suit your vision of what nursing should attempt to be and to do; you might prefer to use parts of different models to illuminate and direct different parts of your vision, or you might be better served by a partially or completely new model of your own devising. Whichever path you choose, it is important to remain true to your own philosophy rather than depart from it for the convenience of using a handy but inappropriate off-the-peg model which will probably impart nuances which your philosophy did not have in its raw state and which you would not wish for your students and patients.

STEP 3   Applying the Nursing Process concept to stabilise the philosophy

You now have a concise package of information conveying your preferred view of what nursing should be like, to guide the curriculum design team in their work. Your concept of the Nursing Process will, of course, further influence the way in which you interpret the activities of nursing practice as you look forward to the next step of listing the tasks entailed in your vision of the nurse's role and function. In fact, the concept of the Nursing Process acts as a firm structure or framework for those tasks as they emerge from the ideals which you have extracted from your earlier discussions; it enables you to grasp more firmly the realities which lie behind the vision. Many other professions are all the poorer for not having the equivalent of our models and process to guide their thinking about practice and preparation for practice.

STEP 4   Listing the tasks of nursing as you have defined it

'Tasks' is a blanket term which covers not only 'things to be done by the application of motor skills' but includes substantial elements of knowledge and the adoption and display of relevant attitudes. For our present purpose, the acquisition of these is also a task. There is no single term in English to cover all these elements; 'skills' is required for the narrower concept of 'motor skills' in manipulating objects, and 'competence', while widely used, has an unfortunate association with the idea of an endowment that is a pittance, barely adequate for the purpose envisaged, but no more.

For this listing it is essential to be guided by the outlines of your philosophy of nursing as it stands at the end of Step 3, interpreted and clarified by the application of a nursing model and the Nursing Process framework. Imagine what tasks the kind of nursing which you have envisaged would entail and then set to work to list them all. This is time-consuming in the extreme but it is a matter upon which it is generally possible to obtain agreement within the team especially if, as seems prudent, you delegate particular areas of nursing practice to be analysed by different members or sub-groups of the team.

The listing of nursing tasks for curriculum design and development is not just *one* way among many others of approaching the operation: it is the only really thorough method, the alternative being the completely student-centred approach outlined in the 'Essential preliminaries' chapter under the sub-heading: 'Why have a curriculum?'. It is still open to you to make the applications of this task analysis more or less student-centred as you wish, by varying the styles of learning, teaching and assessing, but that is another part of the procedure which we shall consider later.

It seems self-evident that the only way to judge success in nurse education is in terms of the efficacy or otherwise of its outcome in the 'tasks' that nurses carry out and the spirit in which they do them. To accept this listing as the basis of the curriculum design procedure is not only to proceed in a soundly 'educational' manner but is also to reassure service staff and prospective students that the gaps sometimes perceived or imagined between the teaching in the schools and the service requirements of the institution will be closed, if they ever existed, by the new curriculum.

The counter-argument, that the students are being prepared in the schools for a long career of problem-solving and decision-making at relatively high levels of administration, though partly true, we hope, is not a completely acceptable reply to young people who suspect that they are destined to spend much of their working lives at the relatively lower levels of the hierarchy and would later be groomed for the higher levels, if selected, by higher-level study elsewhere. It is open to debate, in any case, whether or not the schools can claim to prepare students for more than the first five years or so of their working lives, during which time these intellectually-based craft tasks predominate as the basis of current work and the foundation, if not the substance, of much that is to come.

The difficulty that is almost universally encountered here is to know how detailed to make this listing. Do you specify a task as, for example:

'Prepare a basic dressing trolley setting, prepare the patient for cleaning and dressing a wound and complete the dressing', *or* as something on the lines of:

1. 'Grasp the trolley handle firmly between the thumb and forefinger of the right hand and withdraw it from the parking bay.'
2. 'Turn left and proceed ....'
12, 173 '... Replace the trolley in its parking bay.'

– probably nearer to the former example than to the latter, perhaps finishing up with three or four separate tasks in this instance.

The listing of tasks should be specific, that is, detailed, to the extent that about two hundred and fifty tasks, drawn from the statement of the philosophy of nursing and likely to fall to the lot of a newly-qualified nurse may be identified. Oddly enough, this total seems to be common to a number of similar professions. Since some of these nursing tasks may well be in such ill-defined areas as caring, counselling, educating and so on, it is helpful if they can be defined in terms of some activity or behaviour on the part of the nurse that can be cited as evidence that they are being carried out to an acceptable standard of performance but it is not intended that the strictly measurable 'behavioural' evidence of activity demanded by some educationists should be listed where this would represent a distortion of the nurse's role and function.

At the conclusion of this step it is suggested that you should, for the moment, leave the examination, description and organisation of nursing and turn to consider the nature of the education which you propose for your students, before bringing the two together at a later stage.

STEP 5   Defining the nature of education for nursing: another 'philosophy'

This is a parallel endeavour to the decisions about the nature of nursing which you have just made. It is the other half of the 'education for nursing' equation. You may wish at this stage to be reminded of the distinction that can be drawn between education *in* nursing, a rather bleak, limited and wholly practical approach, and education *for* nursing, an approach which goes beyond the rehearsal of purely practical competences, important as they may be, to produce a person who, as has been already suggested, 'shall be so immersed in nursing that he or she instinctively thinks and acts as a nurse in any conceivable situation where it is appropriate to do so'.

This leads to a further distinction: that between education on the one hand, the process of learning that tends to produce a particular kind of person, and, on the other hand, instruction or training. One should use the term 'education' quite deliberately because the emphasis at the present time and for the foreseeable future, is upon students learning rather than upon teachers teaching, or instructing, or training.

Much modern educational theory and research suggests that students learn best by discovering, researching and creating the important elements of their vocation, as far as is safe and proper and under an agreed level of supervision. This is held to be more stimulating and more likely to result in effective professional performance than being routinely filled up with information and trained to perform tasks carefully and conscientiously but without the opportunity to gain *understanding* by questioning the 'authoritative' sources.

Of course, there are places in the early phases of a nursing curriculum where instruction and training are, perhaps, the most effective ways of promoting certain kinds of essential basic learning before new students acquire 'good' learning habits, but these places may be far fewer, and the period within which they are likely to occur much more limited, than is sometimes realised.

The philosophy of education which is finally adopted should reflect the spirit of the philosophy of nursing which was initially drawn up and which it is intended to impart to students. Your overall aim should probably be to produce qualified nurses who, with no loss of efficiency, can nevertheless consider problems in an objective and clear-sighted manner, accept responsibility, keep their professional skills up-to-date by asking relevant questions and insisting upon satisfactory answers, and seek to promote successful innovations with tact and courtesy.

It is not implied here that you do not already do these things and encourage your students to do them too, but it is important to ensure that students carry on the tradition of doing them in a world where this is becoming increasingly difficult and which will change even more rapidly than our present world is changing now; a world which in the next decade may present them with the most awe-inspiring opportunities and, perhaps, with the most hideous challenges.

The style of the curriculum and of the courses based upon it is a fundamental consideration. Would you wish to attempt to educate and transform students as is urged here, with the attendant accusations of indoctrination, or would you wish to limit your curriculum to one which merely transmits knowledge and skills, and instructs or trains students regardless of their capacity to absorb knowledge, attitudes and skills in the forms in which they might be presented to them? Is the course to be based very firmly within the school or department, or is it to be much more widely involved with the profession and the community? Figure 2.3 shows the diametrically opposed implications of these variables.

You may, of course, decide that different parts of the curriculum require

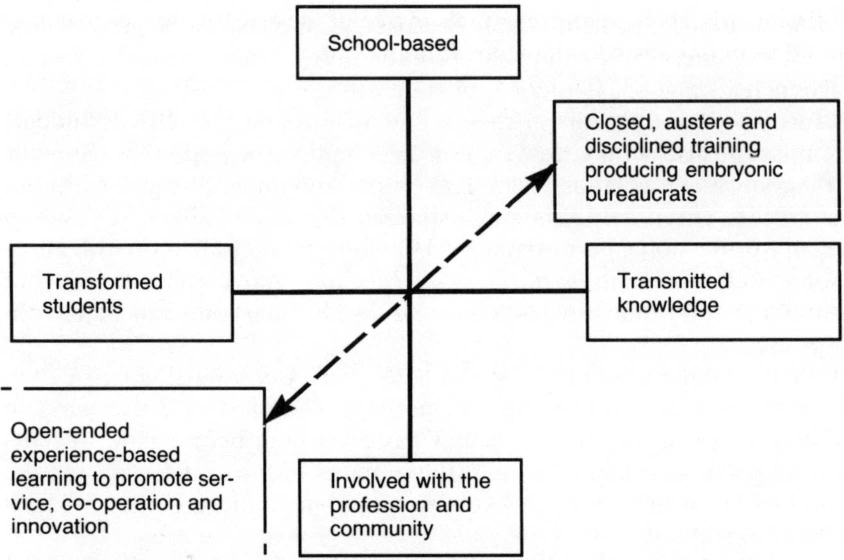

Figure 2.3 The effects of some basic educational decisions in curriculum design and course construction on the future of students and of the profession.

different kinds of treatment along these divergent lines and you should be prepared to cope with the expected problems of either approach.

STEP 6   Defining the categories of knowledge, attitudes and skills available in an educational process

It may come as a surprise that so far there has been no mention of subject content for the curriculum, although we have examined the nature and content of nursing as an abstract idea. Strangely enough, subject content is almost the very last ingredient to be added to the design yet, on reflection, the reason might appear more obvious than one might expect. We are in the business of preparing people of a *particular kind*, rather than people who are possessed solely of a limited body of knowledge or who possess only certain skills, although both knowledge and skills are ultimately of considerable importance. People who are educated to be of a particular kind are distinguished by, and can be identified and assessed by, the fact that they behave in certain effective and economical pre-planned ways when they are faced with given situations. They are quick and resourceful and they get things right first time in their own particular area of expertise. Moreover, they can achieve the same results in relatively unfamiliar circumstances because they are equipped with principles rather than merely with routines;

in other words, they are professionals in one of the few true senses in which the old term has any remaining meaning.

It seems only right, therefore, that the curriculum which prescribes for their education should especially emphasise the cultivation and promotion of certain 'professional' ways of behaving which are important in themselves, to some extent independently of the subject content which is chosen for the exercise and assessment of those ways of behaving. In a rather similar way, nutrition may be regarded as the aim of eating behaviour, the choice of recipes being the last thing to be decided.

The range of the various kinds of knowledge, attitudes and skills which are instrumental in producing certain kinds of behaviour and personality for the occupation of certain roles and the performance of certain professional activities has been identified and is fairly extensive. It has been standardised and listed as a kind of inventory from which particular items can be extracted for each phase of a course of education to assist in producing the required advantages for students. We now have a clear idea of the tasks of nursing, the spirit in which they are to be performed and the spirit in which those who are to perform them are to be prepared. It is time to review the inventory of educational activities and exercises before selecting those which should be most effective in preparing our own students while not robbing them of their autonomy as free and thoughtful individuals.

The list is reproduced in Table 2.1 in an adapted and much abbreviated form in the hope that at this point in the book you will benefit by seeing the full extent of the repertoire. The desired outcomes are listed in the left-hand column and the educational exercises which are known to promote each outcome in the student are shown in the right-hand column. The list is organised into the three sectors of knowledge, attitudes and skills and these have been adapted from the work of the writers to whom they are attributed in the references.

In the next step, to look ahead a little, relevant items from this list are to be selected to assist in the learning and teaching of each nursing task which was identified in Step 4.

STEP 7   Specifying appropriate knowledge, attitudes and skills and educational exercises for each nursing task

It is now necessary for the team to exercise their joint experience in nursing in order to define for each nursing task its main elements and the conditions under which it is normally performed and thence the knowledge, attitudes and skills which a nurse should be able to bring to bear upon its performance in order to define the desired changes in personal attributes. In this way you will set up a series of aims or targets for the students and their teachers and at the same time select outcomes or activities such as analysing and applying

Table 2.1   Table of learning

Knowledge[1]	Column 1	Column 2
The student should:		The student would show mastery of this when she:
1. Know about things:		Distinguishes things from each other
1.1 Terminology		Defines things
1.2 Facts		Recalls facts
1.3 Means of dealing with things		Makes rules for dealing with things
1.4 Conventions		States and describes conventions
1.5 Trends		States and describes trends
1.6 Categories of things		Recognises things as belonging to groups of things
1.7 Criteria for categorising things		Classifies things into groups
1.8 Methods and procedures		States and selects procedures
1.9 Principles and generalisations		Discusses principles
1.10 Theories		States, describes and compares theories
2. Comprehend knowledge		
2.1 Translate ideas		Simplifies ideas in her own words
2.2 Interpret ideas		Demonstrates and explains ideas
2.3 Predict ideas		Infers and predicts on the basis of what is already known
3. Apply knowledge		Applies knowledge to a task
		Revises knowledge for a new situation
		Formulates proposals for development
4. Analyse knowledge		Distinguishes, compares and contrasts elements in a situation, or
		Draws an organisational plan or flow-chart
5. Synthesise knowledge:		
5.1 Produce an original text		Writes a useful summary of a topic derived from various sources
5.2 Produce a plan for action		Writes instructions for carrying out a cooperative procedure
5.3 State the relations in a situation as they are thought to exist		Carries out a minor piece of research and makes a report
6. Evaluate knowledge		Uses external criteria to judge a piece of knowledge as valid or not valid and selects or creates the criteria for judgement
		Criticises constructively and may go on to reconstruct and rearrange that piece of knowledge

Table 2.1 (contd)

Attitudes[2]	Column 1	Column 2
The student should:		The student would show mastery of this when she:
1. Receive (i.e. attend to):		Recognises something (e.g. a problem)
1.1 Become aware of		Takes heed (e.g. of a problem)
1.2 Become willing to pay attention		Shows sensitivity to something
1.3 Control attention		Selects an important element (e.g. a problem), observes it and is able to maintain attention
2. Respond:		
2.1 Acquiesce in making a response		Complies with a request to pay attention and participate
2.2 Become willing to respond		Volunteers to pay attention and to participate
2.3 Find satisfaction in responding		Enjoys the activity of responding; shares it with and recommends it to others
3. Value:		
3.1 Accept the value under consideration		Supports and adheres to, e.g. a belief
3.2 Prefer the value		Chooses this belief above others and prefers it to the state of not having a belief
3.3 Make commitment to the value		Defends it and refutes the opposite belief: works for its acceptance by others
4. Organise values:		
4.1 Conceptualise a value		Analyses ideas and creates a personal statement of the theory behind a belief
4.2 Organise a value system		Places the belief in the context of supporting beliefs and ideas to create a 'way of life'
5. Become characterised by a value or value system		Adopts a belief: changes to conform to it; adheres to it; applies it consistently; evaluates it and if satisfied, resists further change and assumes responsibility for the consequences

Practical skills[3,4]	Column 1	Column 2
The student should:		The student would show mastery of this when she:
1. Exhibit reflex movement		Reacts spontaneously and instinctively to a stimulus
2. Exercise guided manipulation or imitative manipulation		Follows, simulates or copies a task or the steps of a procedure

Table 2.1 (contd)

3. Exercise independent manipulation by trial and error rehearsal	Operates equipment, lifts or turns a patient etc. under supervision only
4. Increase in precision generally Increase in precision of:	Practises to perfection
4.1 Coordination	Synchronises movements
4.2 Sequencing	Performs activities in the right order
4.3 Consistency	Responds regularly and correctly and maintains consistency of output
5. Attain proficiency in:	
5.1 Skill	Performs accurately
5.2 Dexterity	Performs with speed, precision and accuracy
5.3 Acquisition of 'natural' performance	Performs with smoothness, evenness and accuracy
5.4 Automaticity	Performs spontaneously and accurately and with control
6. Adapt by:	
6.1 Improvisation	Overcomes adverse factors by adapting procedures without prior planning
6.2 Modification of environment	Rearranges setting, or –
6.3 Modification of skill	Reorganises skill strategy to overcome adverse factors
7. Experiment and innovate	Tests, develops and implements improved skills, settings, etc. without immediate pressure to adapt Considers whether or not the skilled operation is still valid in the light of new knowledge or changed circumstances

These tabulations have been adapted from the following:

1. Bloom, B.S.., *et al.*, *Taxonomy of educational objectives: classification of educational goals: Handbook I Cognitive domain*, New York, McKay, 1956.
2. Krathwohl, D.R., Bloom, B.S., Masia, B., *Taxonomy of educational objectives: classification of educational goals: Handbook II Affective domain*, New York, McKay, 1964.
3. Simpson, E., *Classification of educational objectives: psychomotor domain*, Urbana, University of Illinois, 1966.
4. Harrow, A.J., *Taxonomy of the psychomotor domain*, New York, McKay, 1972.

knowledge, conceiving and adopting values and gaining skills by which they may be helped to attain them. These aims or targets are so designed within the framework of the curriculum that when students have shown that they have achieved them you can be sure that they have, in the process, acquired and absorbed the knowledge, attitudes and skills that the profession requires of them before they can be recognised as being 'qualified' in that area of the course and the kind of people needed by the profession at that point.

Therefore, it is now your function, in pursuit of this overall end, to decide which of the activities in the left-hand column of the table should be required of students as the necessary contributions to their achievement of each such target which is itself a major contribution to the mastery of a nursing task.

The exercises, success in which is the appropriate and necessary evidence of the mastery of these activities, can then be read off in the right-hand column and may be regarded as forming the framework of the total educational experience which at the end of the course will produce competent nurses with adequate knowledge, attitudes and skills to perform the tasks of nursing to an acceptable standard.

Like some other procedures in curriculum design, this is a long, slow and painstaking operation which seems to soak up endless hours of the team's time, whether they work as a complete committee throughout the procedure or whether sectors of the curriculum's list of tasks are delegated to sub-groups for this part of the operation. There is no quick and easy solution. It must be remembered that within each of the major groups of educational acts in the left-hand column, the individual items of knowledge, attitudes and skills progress from the relatively simple to the very complex. For example, under 'knowledge', distinguishing and defining things and recalling facts are very basic and simple intellectual activities but they must be practised and mastered before the student can go on to such advanced activities as classifying things into groups according to the significant qualities which they possess, analysing them by drawing flow charts of the relationships between them or rearranging their elements into a newly-synthesised piece of original thinking and evaluating it. These latter activities are at the peak of intellectual achievement, but still within the capacity of most of us once we have worked our way up the lower slopes. Therefore, the whole curriculum must be planned as a progression of exercises leading from the simpler kind of activities at the commencement of the course to the more complex activities in its closing stages, in other words a requirement for any higher-level activity at any point in the curriculum assumes the ability on the part of the student to carry out all the preceding lower-level activities in that list.

What we have just discussed are measures to ensure that both students and tutors will be aware of the existence and identity of a series of educational acts or targets that mark the path towards nursing competence and to ensure that both parties will know the nature of the achievements in knowledge, attitudes and practical skills that will signal steady progress through each act on the path, culminating in the desired changes in personal attributes. It will surely come as no surprise to you to discover that each package of a nursing task plus an appropriate act or target to signal mastery of that task plus the activities and the exercises necessary to achieve that act is commonly known as an 'educational objective', although this is the kind of short-hand term which is introduced here only because it is widely used in other books on curriculum design and development.

It is usual to add to the educational objective package a statement as to the set of changes which it is desired to be brought about in the student and the standard to be used to assess the student's achievement of, or failure to achieve, the objective and to master the task. Here is an example of a nursing task and its related educational objective package to clarify the nature of this most significant 'building brick' in a curriculum:

> Task: 'To prepare a basic dressing trolley and prepare the patient for dressing a wound'.

> Educational objective for the achievement of this learning:
> While under the supervision of a tutor or clinical teacher in the practice ward, the student will state clearly the reasons for the procedure; will select and lay out on the top and bottom trays of the trolley as appropriate the full range of necessary basic items; will prepare the 'patient' by explaining the procedure, screening, positioning and reassuring the 'patient' and exposing the dressing site. Changes sought: to plan and execute procedures with care. This task will be assessed by the supervisor who will award one mark for each item or part of the procedure correctly dealt with up to a maximum of 25 marks. Marks will be deducted at the rate of one per minute for time spent on the procedure in excess of 10 minutes. A score of 20 marks or more will be regarded as evidence of success at this stage of the course.

In order to obtain some idea as to how this might be translated into actual academic exercises in the 'class-room', you might find it useful to note that the principal relevant *activities* from the Table might be as follows:

> Knowledge: of things (1.2), facts (1.2), conventions (1.4), methods and procedures (1.8), application of knowledge (3)
> The student can identify the trolley and its contents, recall and apply the knowledge of the conventional layout and the procedures of laying out the trolley and preparing the 'patient'.

> Attitudes: controlling attention (1.3), making commitment to a value (3.3)
> The student can concentrate on the task in hand and feel a determination to ensure the comfort and well-being of the patient committed to her care.

> Skills: attainment of proficiency and dexterity (5.2), improvisation (6.1)
> The student should exhibit, at this stage of the course, a reasonable degree of dexterity in handling the equipment and the patient and should be able to improvise a solution to problems created by an unsatisfactory environment, for example, poor light or an over-crowded ward.

The exercises listed in the right-hand column of the tables against these activities, or at least an appropriate selection of them, would then be woven into the lessons planned in Step 8 to teach this task, with the virtual assurance that if the curriculum be well-designed the successful student would be both competent in preparing the trolley and patient and would also be the best kind of person to accompany a real patient through a possibly distressing experience. It should be further noted that the successful mastery of a complicated task often has to be accomplished by the simultaneous achievement of a number of converging educational objectives. On the other hand, several different tasks may sometimes be served by the achievement of a single, carefully-formulated educational objective, thus leading to economies in time and resources.

These lists of the educational objectives for education for nursing, once completed with their accompanying specifications of the elements of knowledge, attitudes and skills required for their achievement, must now be examined and edited to eliminate overlap and inconsistencies and to take advantage of opportunities for economies such as those suggested above. You may integrate them into one list and perhaps summarise them in order to bring them within a reasonable compass. You should publicise the list and check it with everyone in the service sector who may be concerned with students and their learning and perhaps modify it in accordance with any reasonable suggestions which might be made in those quarters.

It cannot be sufficiently stressed that while the declared tasks of nursing and the broad aims of education for nursing may be of widespread, almost universal, validity within the culture or country in which they were conceived, the educational objectives which are derived from them, the planned outcome of each course, module or even single lesson, are produced for a known group of students in a particular institution. They should not be specified for other students elsewhere unless this is the policy of the profession as a whole or its governing body. Nevertheless, they should be framed so as to produce a qualified nurse who is immediately recognisable to the discerning eye as a professional in her own right in almost any circumstances and they may reasonably be tested in other institutions.

STEP 8   Allocating subject content and methods of learning, teaching and assessing to lesson units

So far learning has been described only in terms of the desirable attributes, acts, objectives and exercises to be specified for the mastery of each nursing task, the purpose being not to fill a pint pot with a quart of facts and purely manual skills, but to produce a special kind of person by putting her through a process of genuine education. Subject matter has not been discussed in detail but has, of course, been implied in the discussion of nursing tasks, each task necessarily having a specified area of interest, procedures and links with other elements and areas of the nursing activity.

Once you have produced a well-integrated framework of educational objectives and their associated learning experiences from the table in Step 7, each objective must be invested with its carefully chosen subject content (at last!) in this closing stage of the design process. The long list which is created at this point can then be broken down into modules and individual lesson units as appropriate for the needs and conditions of each school or department.

It may be extremely useful to identify at this point a core of nursing knowledge, attitudes, skills and essential basic activities which is virtually universal and even shared by other professionals in paramedical sectors. You may do this in the form of a diagram as suggested in Figure 2.4. You can then concentrate your resources upon this and relegate more specialised and less essential, but still interesting, topics to a separate part of the course or regard them as a range of 'optional extras' from which the student can make a choice according to her interests. The core could thus be regarded as a foundation course: a preparation for a later career in some area other than nursing and, in a sense, beyond general nursing, such as school nursing,

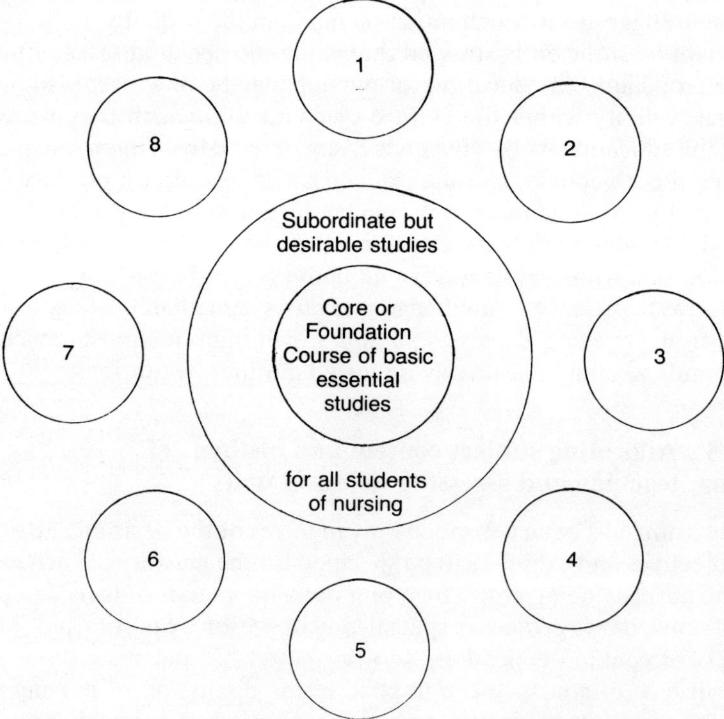

Items 1–8 are specialised or general interest topics, perhaps offered as 'optional extras', to cater for the special interests of some or all students of nursing.

Figure 2.4 The 'core' curriculum concept.

occupational health nursing or some other speciality as well as, primarily, in general nursing itself.

It is also sometimes advantageous to take important core topics and, while teaching their basic elements early in the course, return to deal with them in greater detail or from different points of view as the students' understanding increases as they progress up the resulting curriculum 'spiral' (see Figure 2.5).

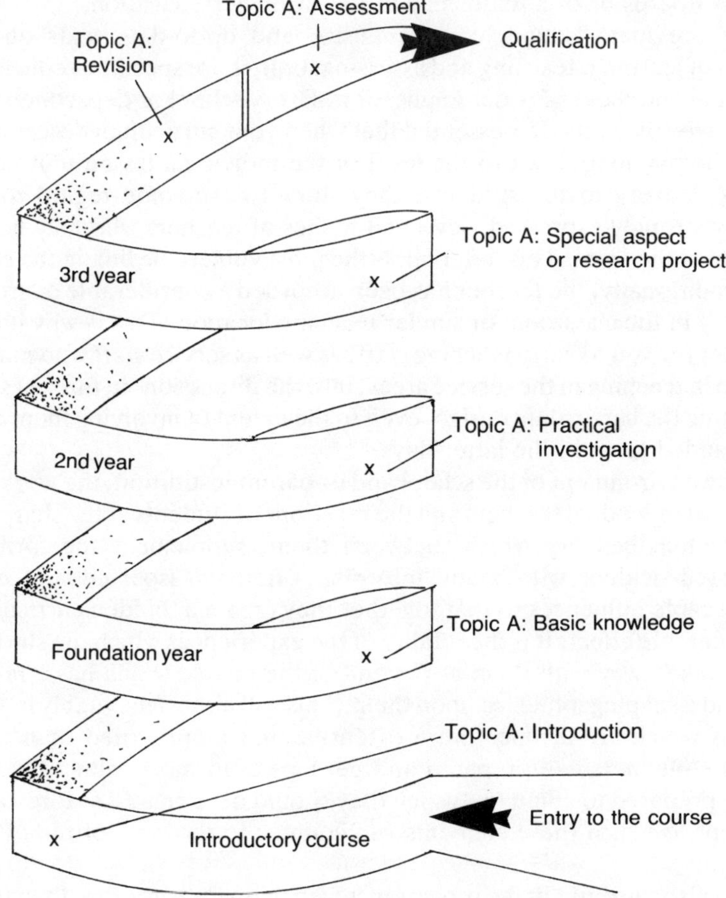

Figure 2.5 The 'spiral' curriculum concept.

It is also time for you to consider and allocate to these lesson units an indication of appropriate learning and teaching methods and to identify means of assessing whether or not objectives have been achieved by students at each successive level of lessons, modules and of the course as a whole. As in the case of the educational objectives, it would be wrong for an outsider to attempt to specify subject content, structure, learning and teaching methods and systems of assessment for students he does not know. These all depend to a large extent upon the outlook, facilities, time and human resources of each individual school and its parent institution, especially where the latter may be a university or polytechnic as opposed to a hospital. Perhaps the only extent to which these are not decided by local people in the light of local conditions is the extent to which they are subject to the requirements of the National Boards or of a major institution of higher education.

There are many sound, comprehensive and up-to-date texts on the methods of learning, teaching and assessing, both those specific to education for nursing and those of wider application. Every school or department has its own favourite texts. It is essential that when your curriculum design team carries the planning down to the level of the individual lesson unit at the point of delivery to the students, they should have some regard to the probably strongly expressed views and wishes of teachers who may not be members of the team. This, after all, is the most vulnerable link in the chain since, traditionally, the teacher has been accorded a considerable degree of autonomy in the classroom or similar teaching location. This is why it is so important for you to carry teaching staff, as well as service staff who may be involved in teaching in the service areas, into the discussions in this last stage of planning the curriculum design, even to the extent of involving them *all* in the expanded team in the latter days.

It is the environment of the school and its parent institution, the work and attitudes of individual teachers and the reactions of students at the sharp end of curriculum delivery which, between them, supplement the formally planned curriculum with many informal, often unsuspected and quite unforeseeable influences so that together they create a 'hidden curriculum' of considerable effect. It is the totality of the experiences which the students actually take away with them at the end of the course which has a lasting effect and a shaping influence upon them. This will almost inevitably include elements which are at once more extensive and more varied than those which the planners had prepared and perhaps even more influential than they are prepared to admit but which they should be prepared to forestall to the extent to which these elements run counter to the aims of the official curriculum.

This is also the point in the process at which many factors other than those already dealt with must be planned in accordance with the availability of resources in your school. These include equipment, rooms, timetables, support staff and a host of other facilities. Everything which influences students, however remotely, is part of the curriculum, overt or hidden, right through to the comfort of their rooms in the residences. In particular, sound and comprehensive library and information services are crucial to success.

The selection of students for the re-designed course must also be discussed since you may well decide that it makes sense to select those most likely to live up to your philosophy of nursing and profit from your philosophy of education for nursing even if it means subjecting them to simple but reliable psychological tests in addition to the usual interviews prior to acceptance.

STEP 9 Validating, presenting and implementing the completed curriculum

After the relief and exultation of the completion of the curriculum has subsided, it is desirable to review the whole construction, moving back up the process from the arrangements for the individual lessons right back to the philosophies of education and nursing in order to make sure that the latter have been followed closely, and to ensure that the educational experiences can be delivered in the school or department and that they cover all the desirable educational objectives in sufficient strength and variety to enable your students to achieve those objectives with a high likelihood of success.

You should make a further check through the process, this time in order to ensure, as far as possible, that the experiences provided are such as to change a high proportion of the persons who live and work through them into 'the kind of person who is so immersed in nursing that he or she instinctively thinks and acts as a nurse in any conceivable situation in which it is appropriate to do so'. You may add the provision that the nurse so educated can be guaranteed to perform tasks of nursing competently and in the spirit of the philosophy of nursing which you drafted at the beginning of the process as the key to the whole design. If it appears that this will, indeed, be the case, all else being equal, then you can regard the curriculum as having been validated; that is, you are satisfied that it can do, in theory at least, what it was designed to do.

The preparation and presentation of the actual curriculum document is in itself a major editing and publishing feat, for the full statement and detailed specification of a curriculum is of considerable length with many sections to cover all the above operations as well as sections for the major elements required for the special approval of the accrediting body, whether it is a National Board or a university or polytechnic governing body. The actual launching of the new curriculum may, perhaps, be best described as a 'heart-stopping anti-climax': only the most outrageous paradox can describe the feelings of the now unoccupied members of your design team as they prowl empty corridors and listen to the tomb-like silence that lies behind closed classroom doors where their 'baby' has been delivered into the hands of others.

But this, of course, is only a temporary respite!

STEP 10 Reviewing, revising and re-validating the curriculum: evaluation

Success will be confirmed or disproved by careful monitoring of the curriculum during the first complete course to be delivered under its control. You must base this evaluation upon what is found to happen during every minute of every day, not just on the day that examination results are announced. Teething troubles with regard to new subject content, new learning, teaching and assessment methods, inappropriate timing and inadequately briefed teachers must be eliminated daily without losing sight of the grand design. At the end of the course you must rigorously inspect the grand design itself for major flaws and continuing relevance to changing conditions in practice and in the profession generally. This must be done at the end of *every* course and at any interim point where major weaknesses are suspected. This should be done preferably by the members of your original team with only a leavening of new members who are being groomed to take over the work of development in due course.

Like the traveller who encountered the Old Man of the Sea, you will never get the curriculum off your back, but this martyrdom will be for the greater good of present colleagues and future generations of nurses. This will be your consolation – and your epitaph!

Chapter 3

Introduction to a closer study of the curriculum design and development procedure: curriculum models

The intention in the remaining part of this book is to supplement the preceding outline of the complete curriculum design and development procedure with a series of extensive explanatory footnotes, one for each step of the process, which should provide you with a fairly detailed analysis of the sources, nature and purpose of each step and some idea as to its construction and overall contribution to the growing curriculum structure.

All these steps have been briefly described already in quite practical terms in the outline but here is an opportunity to adjourn regularly to a more discursive treatment, to follow up just a few references which are almost certain to be in the stock of your hospital, school or department library. You may also like to consider from time to time, the implications of the decisions which you are called upon to make and of any doubts and diversions which you might be tempted to entertain. In the meantime, however, you might consider it appropriate to review some systems of curriculum design, or the models which represent them; yes, curriculum designers have models too.

A curriculum model, rather like a nursing model or a model in any other sphere of intellectual activity, is simply an organised set of ideas or concepts (hence 'conceptual model') which displays in words or diagrams the essential features of a proposed venture, stripped of all the complications which tend to obscure its distinguishing features in a full-scale theoretical explanation or practical demonstration. You might wish to consider briefly why this particular model is being recommended as opposed to some of the others which are available. The various systems fall into two major groups which are commonly characterised as 'product models' and 'process models' respectively, although it would be more accurate to describe them as two opposed positions at either end of the same spectrum: the basic curriculum structure which is described in this book.

The 'product' systems tend to be defined by the fairly precise setting of educational aims and objectives, as we have seen, by the formal design, organisation and testing of learning experiences for the students and by the design and implementation of methods whereby the students' achievement of the original aims and objectives can be virtually assured and their degree of success measured with an acceptable accuracy by the teacher.

As already suggested, this system envisages as its 'product' a competent nurse, produced to a known and mutually agreed specification. It is, to that extent, a relatively efficient and relatively economical system in a sector of society that is usually short of resources of all kinds. It offers the students a predictable programme and constant support by reducing unknown factors to the unavoidable minimum of a residual hidden curriculum. It is a cohesive and adaptable system which can be applied at any level of education and to courses of any length or complexity and which can accommodate a wide variety of approaches to the learning of knowledge, behaviour and skills. It is the system favoured and demonstrated in this book and is sometimes variously referred to as the 'systematic', 'objectives' or 'behavioural' curriculum model.

It earned a quite unjustified reputation as an instrument for indoctrination when applied with excessive rigour and some misunderstanding of its limitations by some of the early pioneers of the 'programmed learning' method of self-instruction in the 1960s. The 'product' model has been criticised, in particular, as tending to promote short-term and relatively trivial outcomes in rather narrow fields of study, and of promoting 'information-gathering' as opposed to 'discovering' and 'experiencing'. It is said that objectives are likely to be so numerous and so difficult to define in many cases as to render the process unmanageable and it is also said that it is difficult, if not impossible, to specify what the student 'should' learn and often undesirable to attempt to do so when learning might be better if left open-ended. Critics add that it is wrong to fragment learning into the separate sectors of knowledge, behaviour and skills. Above all it has been condemned because it is said that the system depends upon identifying measurable behaviour on the part of the student as a sign that any learning has taken place at all and for some people this seems to be too reminiscent of early experiments with rats and pigeons.

If, after reading this catalogue of criticisms, you believe that you are about to back the wrong horse, consider each criticism in turn once more. Try to determine for yourself, in the light of what you already know of the curriculum design process from the preceding outline, to what extent each criticism is a criticism, not of the method itself, but of the way in which the method could be carelessly, incompetently or even maliciously applied by the wrong kind of educator. Consider how easily these undesirable characteristics could be avoided or eliminated if, in fact, anybody were ever tempted to incorporate them into a curriculum in the first place.

Opponents, those who would seek to promote various 'process' models, emphasise the importance of the opposite virtues; of students achieving more extensive and lasting gains when they are permitted to identify and pursue their own learning needs within a very wide field of objectives anticipated, as far as possible, by the curriculum designer; of students gaining invaluable experience of the real world by constructing solutions to problems which they identify or which are brought to their attention; and of students developing and exploring their own potential and pursuing their own range of interests through strategies of their own devising. It is said that in a process model, 'intentions' replace 'objectives' and that, just as in the Nursing Process, the student, rather than the tutor, learns to assess, plan, implement and evaluate her work with minimal formal supervision. In fact, in one process model, that proposed by Stenhouse, the teacher becomes a neutral chairman or fellow-researcher alongside the students in the classroom. In particular an 'experiential taxonomy' has been proposed by Steinaker and Bell which not only offers the student learning-through-experience over the widest possible range of learning and teaching methods, but leads the student to absorb gradually, and later exhibit, the results of the experience in her behaviour, culminating in the admirable objective, or intention, of disseminating the results of her experiential learning as an exemplar and role model to her colleagues and later, perhaps, as a teacher of students in her turn.

Looking back again at all that has been said about the design of curricula so far in this book, consider how all these desirable features of the 'process' could, and indeed should, be built into the basic curriculum structure represented by the so-called 'product' model to varying degrees as might be considered appropriate for various groups of students in various schools and departments. If this is conceded, one might suggest that since this curriculum is intended for use in a vital and demanding public service profession and administered within a system of higher vocational education, both of which are accountable ultimately to the public and to the public purse, we should look for a product of predictable and consistent quality at a predictable cost. These are the attendant advantages of a planned learning situation which were outlined under the heading, 'Why have a curriculum?'.

In any case, it is commonly observed that a process model, however liberal in theory, often turns out to be remarkably like a product model in practice. The process is rather a way of applying certain desirable features to a basic curriculum structure than a curriculum structure in its own right.

Having cleared the ground somewhat, you may feel ready now to take a closer look at the first step on the road towards a curriculum structure in the next section. In doing this you might wish to seek the help of an expert consultant in curriculum design. It is usual to distinguish five phases of a consultancy: defining the function of the consultant and negotiating a contract; assessing and analysing the problems; assigning the priorities and resources and setting up intermediate objectives; developing the skills of the client while jointly pursuing the objectives; and providing follow-up evaluation and support.

The consultant may take the initiative or may prefer to remain in the background as an observer and advise only when the need for further information and resources becomes apparent, leaving the client to assume overall responsibility for the establishment of aims and the direction of the procedure. This would appear to be more in accord with the ethics of the consultative role. The consultant should have a good working knowledge of nursing and its professional setting, education theory, group processes and communication and, of course, research methods. Rather significantly, it is assumed that a consultant investigating a nursing curriculum would normally choose to adopt what is referred to in the article as the 'broad and comprehensive...' product or objectives model as a firmer base for curriculum analysis and construction than that offered by the relatively imprecise and less predictable nature of the process model.

Further reading

Heath, Jean, *Curriculum design in nursing: a practical guide for course planners* Sheffield, English National Board Learning Resources Unit, 1982.
A helpful and pleasantly discursive treatment of the procedure.
Kenworthy, Neil, Nicklin, Peter, A taxonomy for the curriculum *Senior Nurse*, March 1986, Vol. 4, No. 3, pp. 11–14.
Use of the experiential taxonomy at North Lincolnshire School of Nursing.
Marks-Maran, Diane, Challenge of change *Senior Nurse*, September 1986, Vol. 5, No. 3, pp. 32–33.
A plea for experiential, reflective and counselling approaches to the nursing curriculum.
Pointon, Harold, Jumping off the band-wagon *Nursing times*, 28 August 1985, Vol. 81, No. 35, pp. 43–45.
An alternative to the product model, dealing especially with the teacher as a classroom researcher/chairman.
Quinn, F. M., *Principles and practice of nurse education* London, Croom Helm, 1980.
Raichura, Liz, Using the objectives model (of curriculum design) *Nursing Times*, 10 June 1987, Vol. 83, No. 23, (QUEST SUPPLEMENT) pp. 59–60.
Sheehan, John, Curriculum models: product versus process *Journal of Advanced Nursing*, November 1986, Vol. 11, No. 6, pp. 671–678.
Steinaker, N., Bell, R., *The experiential taxonomy: a new approach to teaching and learning* New York, Academic Press, 1979.

Stenhouse, Lawrence, *Introduction to curriculum research and development* London, Heinemann, 1975 (reprinted 1984).
An easily read standard book on the subject, although largely confined to the school curriculum in general education.
Wheeler, D. K., *Curriculum process* London, University of London Press, 1967.
A long but lucid account of curriculum design, closely reasoned in a scholarly manner.

If you decide to engage outside assistance in the work of curriculum design it might be helpful to read:

Sanders, Louise *et al.*, Curriculum consultant, would you help us out?... practical guidelines for analyzing a nursing curriculum and an introducton to the consultative intervention *Nursing and Health Care*, June 1981, Vol. 2, No. 6, pp. 315–321.

Step 1 Defining the nature of nursing: a 'philosophy'

Reminder

The *objects* of making a philosophy are:

- To define the nature of the vocation for which students are to be educated and thereby shape the future of the profession.
- To define an ideal, with positive views on clients' needs, what a nurse should do and, above all, what she should be.
- To draw from the philosophy all the requirements for a curriculum to produce such a person.

The *method* of making a philosophy is to identify and define the key ideas about nursing and incorporate them into a brief philosophical statement about its nature and purpose.

The word 'philosophy' is used here with some reluctance because while we all believe we know exactly what it means, we still suspect that it is a thinly-disguised trap for the unwary and that there lurks behind the word a much more demanding and potentially embarrassing involvement with the subject of the philosophical enquiry than we may care to accept. The dictionary definitions are, as one might expect, clear and reassuring:

> The love, study or pursuit of... knowledge of things and their causes, whether theoretical or practical; the knowledge or study of the principles of human action or conduct... that department of knowledge or study which deals with ultimate reality... the study of the principles of some particular branch of knowledge, experience or activity. ... (*Oxford universal dictionary*, 3rd edn, 1944, revised by C. T. Onions from the text prepared by W. Little, H. W. Fowler and J. Coulson)

We who 'love, study and pursue knowledge' about nursing are simply asked for our views about:

- The 'theoretical and practical nature' of nursing, its origins and purposes.
- The 'principles' which we believe should guide its members in their efforts to carry out such 'human' (and humane) 'actions' as are required in their efforts to become the kind of people who are recognisably nurses because of their 'conduct'.
- The 'ultimate reality' which lies behind the aims and endeavours of the nursing profession.
- The nature of the 'particular principles' which distinguish nursing from all other similar activities.

In order to assemble such an informed set of views we firstly need to define for ourselves a particular viewpoint or stance, a perspective or direction in which to gaze and some idea of what we are looking for – a goal or purpose for nursing – upon which to focus our vision. These matters may be intensely private and personal parts of our professional lives and we may be reluctant to speak about them, but if a nurse does not have some inkling of her own viewpoint, perspective and goal, however vague and ill-defined, she is to that extent less than a full professional. She might, then, drift towards a depersonalised and, perhaps, uncritical acceptance of the existing situation and she is likely to make a contribution that lacks zest and dedication.

The historical background

To be fully conscious of these matters in this way is to have a 'philosophy' and therefore to be in a position to make a supremely worthwhile contribution to the profession; zestful and dedicated.

Over the period of the last century or so we have been reminded that this outlook is as valid for a group as it is for a single individual. Florence Nightingale laboured as an individual to extract secular nursing from its unsavoury past against the deadweight of general apathy, broken fitfully by opposition in some quarters, as she sought to bring about sufficient improvement in the generally squalid physical environment of the sick to allow nature a fair chance to effect its own cure. Her task analysis of nursing became the 'syllabus' for 'training' until comparatively recently. For half a century after her death, except for short periods of crisis in the two World Wars, the profession as a group tended to relapse into the same uncritical acceptance of the existing situation which is referred to above and, it seems, with the same result: a general lack of corporate zest and dedication in the absence of a widely-held professional philosophy.

The existing situation, seemingly immutable, was a blend of traditional values such as asceticism and humility, which contributed to the perpetuation of an image of the nurse as accepting or even seeking an almost superhuman degree of self-discipline and self-denial in pursuit of an over-riding duty to her patients and her professional superiors. Such a nurse was expected to spurn the quest for the improvement of her very poor pay and conditions of work and to be concerned less with the actual acquisition of nursing knowledge, attitudes and skills than with the opportunity to 'care' in general terms. One suspects that this was the outlook of Emily, Viscountess Strangford, who sought only a relatively brief period of hospital training for her ladies and seemed not to envisage their making a career, much less a living, out of their calling.

There was, too, a substantial element of romanticism in the way in which the difficult, down-to-earth search for truth in matters of the human condition – anatomy and physiology, clinical disease and injury, public health and social reality – gave way for several decades to a vague idealism. Visions of what could, and should, be the nature of nursing were diverted towards the vision of the 'Lady of the Lamp', which the Lady herself would probably have found unacceptable in her mature years, and towards that of the subservient nurse who should feel a warm glow of satisfaction in sacrificing herself to the needs of others. In particular, she was expected to serve the requirements of the physicians and surgeons and their medical models of diagnosis and treatment, and the needs of the patient in his capacity as the embodiment of a disease or injury.

Gradually, it seems, there emerged from the unspeakable horrors of the two World Wars and their accompanying massive problems for nurses on both the military and civilian fronts in Europe and the Far East, two new strands to replace the outworn and now untenable values of asceticism, humility, self-sacrifice and self-effacement. In those circumstances, over-worked and under-equipped, nurses realised that they had perforce to undertake genuine and inescapable responsibilities and that, in the words of E. O. Bevis, 'truth is whatever works in the given circumstances'.[1] Their new-found pragmatism, still serving the medical model and remaining focused on the disease or injury, the 'appendectomy in Bed 7', led indirectly to the fragmentation of the nursing body into an increased number of specialisms. Many of the new activities were lost irrevocably to nursing but at the same time some new areas of knowledge and skill were opened up for them out of what remained of their former functions as a result of new understandings and new techniques.

During the last twenty or thirty years, there has been a slow but unmistakable change in outlook and the emergence of a positive, shared philosophy created by nurses for their own guidance. This appeared to involve some redefinition of the basic values of nursing practice, revolving around the issues of the client, the environment, an acceptable quality of life and the true nature of caring. There was a new view of the uniqueness and innate worth of each and every human being, regardless of his or her condition and circumstances. The 'holistic' view was that a person amounts to more than the mere sum of his or her physical parts and should be nursed accordingly with respect and consultation. There was a requirement that the nurse should seek to promote the client's health and capacity to care for himself, to communicate effectively, to coordinate the work of others towards a common goal in a team approach and to tend, protect and treat those who for the time being lack the capacity to care for themselves. There was a new appreciation of the need for constant research and renewal guided by the application of nursing models and the nursing process to these activities (see Figure 4.1).

Finally, there has been a growing conviction of the need for the nurse to be an active member of her professional association and to render herself personally and, in cooperation with her colleagues, collectively accountable for all that she and her unified profession undertake and achieve. A fundamental change of attitudes was required on every hand.

Some important documents

This awakening of recent decades is reflected stage by stage in the unfolding literature of the period and some of the landmarks of this literature are reviewed below. It is, perhaps, no coincidence that the process appeared to begin after the turmoil and total disruption of the two wars and the brief, uneasy period of so-called peace that separated them. The impetus for change might well have been the United Nations General Assembly's 'Universal declaration of human rights', adopted on 10 December 1948 by forty-eight votes to none, with eight abstentions by the Communist countries and South Africa and Saudi Arabia.[2] Article 1 states unequivocally that:

> All human beings are born free and equal in dignity and rights. They are endowed with reason and conscience, and should act towards one another in a spirit of brotherhood.

Twenty-nine other articles set out a catalogue of these rights in all spheres of life: under the law, within the family unit, as a social, spiritual, political and wage-earning person, entitled to peace, education and health care. In respect of the latter, Article 25 provides that:

1. Everyone has the right to a standard of living adequate for the health and well-being of himself and his family, including food, clothing, housing and medical care and necessary social services...
2. Motherhood and childhood are entitled to special care and assistance...

The declaration was implemented under the terms of three International Covenants in 1976 and 1979, by which time much of the spadework of implementation in the widening circle of consenting countries had already

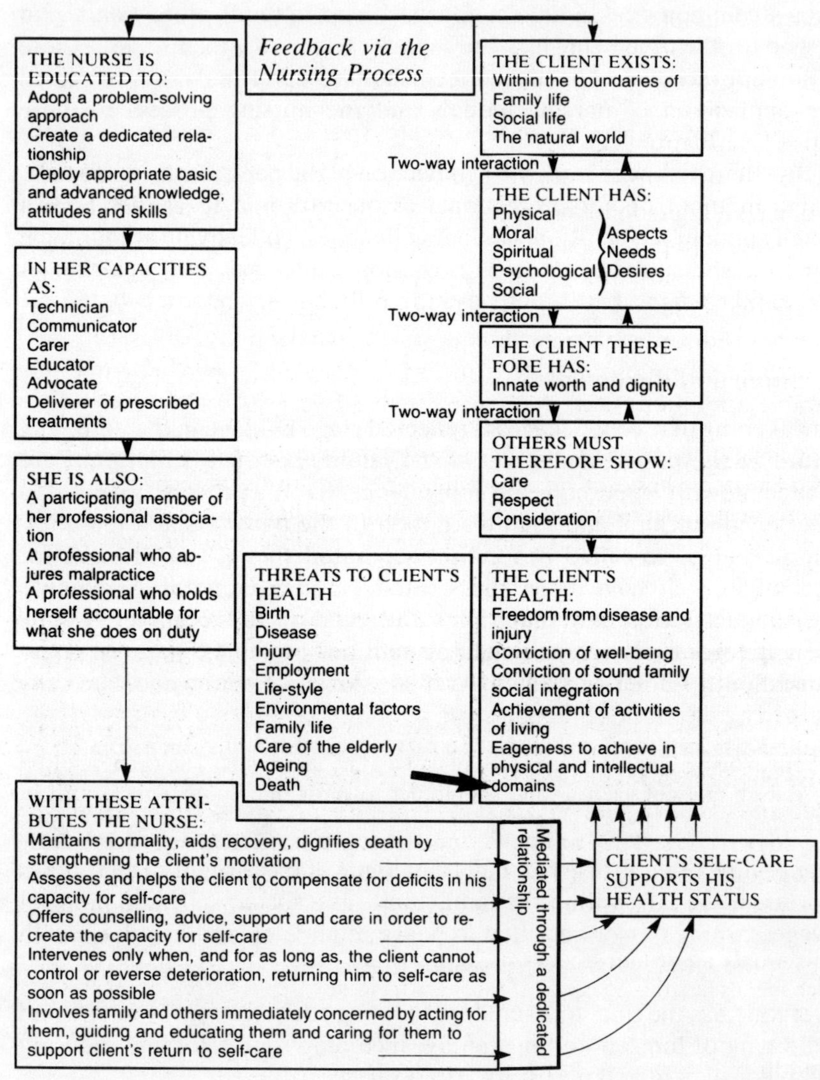

Figure 4.1 A conceptual map of the model of nursing.

been done. In the course of this spadework, Virginia Henderson had, in 1960 and again in 1969, clarified some 'Basic principles of nursing care'[3] on behalf of the Geneva-based International Council of Nurses. This had gone through eleven reprints before the last of the International Covenants had been ratified and its importance had been signalled by the quotation in the foreword from the World Health Organization's Expert Committee on Nursing in its 'Report of the first session, February 1950'[4]:

> In many countries where medicine is highly developed and nursing is not, the health status of the people does not reflect the advanced stage of medicine.

Virginia Henderson starts from the premise that the nurse has been regarded in the popular imagination, as a person with a role that changes so rapidly over a period of time and in response to the many varying circumstances of the client and the society in which he lives, that it is extraordinarily difficult to produce a satisfactorily comprehensive definition of her role, still less an adequate philosophy. She concludes, in a well-known but eminently repeatable quotation, that:

> The unique function of the nurse is to assist the individual, sick or well, in the performance of those activities contributing to health or its recovery (or to a peaceful death) that he would perform unaided if he had the necessary strength, will or knowledge. And to do this in such a way as to help him gain independence as rapidly as possible.

The activities concerned, such as breathing, eating, eliminating, communicating, worshipping, working, playing and learning, are listed, but circumstances both personal and pathological such as age, mental state and shock, are held to render the planning and implementation of nursing care an applied art rather than a matter of routine. In particular, she is concerned that the client who is capable of making choices about his care should be enabled and encouraged to make informed choices and that these should be respected, the nurse acting independently only in matters in which the client cannot express an informed choice and in which the medical staff do not make a formal prescription. In those circumstances:

> she can only assist him (the client) in those activities contributing to that state which means health – to *him* – or recovery from disease – to *him* – or what is – to *him* – a good death.

In addition, the nurse helps the client to carry out the therapy recommended by the medical staff and gives support to, and receives support from the members of the team to which she belongs.

This document was followed, in 1973, by the 'International code of nursing ethics' promulgated by the International Nursing Council's Council of International Representatives at a meeting in Mexico City.[5] Its importance, clarity and conciseness are such that it is in almost universal use as the basis of a philosophy of nursing. The document stresses the fundamental responsibilities of the nurse:

> to promote health, to prevent illness, to restore health and alleviate suffering.

Inherent in nursing is:

> respect for the life, dignity and rights of man. It is unrestricted by considerations of nationality, race, creed, colour, sex, politics or social status.

Nurses render health services to those who require nursing care, to the individual, the family and the community, and seek to promote an environment in which the values, customs and spiritual beliefs of the individual are respected. His personal confidences are to be shared with others, subject to his approval, only when absolutely necessary to his well-being. The nurse holds herself responsible for her own competence and that of her team, works to the highest standards and maintains similarly high standards of personal and professional conduct, whether practising or carrying out such activities as teaching, researching or participating in the promotion of adequate working conditions for herself and her colleagues.

Four subsequent documents have gone some way towards forging the link between the idealism of a pure nursing philosophy and the realities of clinical practice. Three of them are Royal College of Nursing discussion documents: 'Standards of nursing care', 1980 and 'Towards standards', 1981, the interim and second reports of the R.C.N. Working Committee on Standards of Nursing Care (England and Wales)[6,7] and 'Standards of care in psychiatric nursing practice', 1986.[8] In the two former cases the Committee began with an attempt to identify factors that could be used to measure professionally acceptable standards of nursing care but it soon became inescapably preoccupied with analysing the role of the nurse, together with the supplementary roles of nurse educators and nurse managers. In the event the function of 'assisting sick people with the activities of daily living' was reiterated as the focus of nursing work, together with the complementary work of teaching the client and his supporting group how to manage the changed situation that comes with later independence. The general role, especially the central role of the generalist ward-sister/charge nurse, was emphasised at the expense of the roles of the specialist nurses such as psychotherapists and stomatherapists and a possible area of conflict between the two elements was highlighted.

The outward and visible evidence of an acceptable philosophy of nursing in these circumstances was held to be two-fold: on the one hand the objective, observable and, in some cases, measurable, behaviour of nurses, framed in the pattern of the nursing process and, on the other hand, the actual products of nursing in terms of equally objective, observable and measurable benefits for the clients. Measurement, to be of use, must obviously be made against standards which are generally acceptable and must take account of the nursing environment with its personnel management policies, available resources and so on.

Among the eight key factors which were specified as prerequisites for the professional control of nursing standards, the first to be listed was 'a philosophy of nursing', preceding such factors as knowledge and skills, autonomy, accountability, resource-control, organisation and management, relationships with other professionals, especially doctors, and the management of change. Regarding the matter of a philosophy, the second report said:

> This term is used, loosely, to refer to the beliefs and values that every nurse holds about what nursing is and what it is for. In our first report we identified three component parts: a concept that 'nursing' is a particular and identifiable approach to patient care which is distinct from that of... any other discipline... in which the patient is central as a whole person and as a unique individual. Nursing's aim, usually, is to define goals with, and for, the patient towards the achievement of those activities of daily living which ensure the patient's maximum independence. There are circumstances when, at best, the patient's independence is limited. Here, the nurse must ensure that the patient or his relatives have knowledge of, and access to, all agencies that exist to provide the support needed...

The report concludes, pessimistically, and with a certain coyness, that 'It is not yet typical for everyone to see nursing in this way', but it looks to the day when this philosophy will generate commitment at all levels of practice, education and management.

The fourth document which you should consider in this step of the process is the UKCC's 'Code of professional conduct for the nurse, midwife and health visitor', 2nd edition, 1984,[9] the slim red pamphlet which is subject to periodic review and open to suggestions and comments from those for whose guidance it is issued. In fourteen brief paragraphs on two centre-spread pages, it sums up virtually everything that has been said over the last thirty years about:

1. Safeguarding the well-being of clients under the nurse's care.
2. Ensuring the safety of clients from her actions or failure to act.
3. Improving her professional knowledge.
4. Acknowledging her own limitations.
5. Working in collaboration with others.
6. Taking account of the customs and beliefs of clients.
7. Acknowledging her own conscientious objection to some aspects of practice.
8. Avoiding abuse of the nurse-client relationship.
9. Respecting the client's confidences.
10. Ensuring the best feasible environment and resources for the client.

11. Safeguarding good working practices and avoiding overloading colleagues.
12. Assisting colleagues to improve their knowledge and competence.
13. Refusing favours or bribes.
14. Refusing to allow her name or position to be used to promote any activity which might appear to prejudice her independence.

Some concepts for your own philosophy of nursing

If you should wish to replace, or supplement, this considerable body of professional lore with a completely fresh and original philosophy of your own devising, there is absolutely no reason why you should not do so. You should, however, be aware of the dangers of losing contact with your roots in a developing body of thought and you should be confident in detecting and giving appropriate weight to the main ideas which, in your view, permeate nursing and need to be taken into account in your curriculum. You may decide that, since disease and injury appear to be no longer the central focus of nursing but are regarded primarily as obstacles to a full and normal life, the central issues could be considered along something like the following lines:

1. Man: a natural, holistic living system with freedom of choice but accountable for his actions and his influence upon the environment to his conscience and to the rules of his society.
2. Society: a set of conventions for the protection, nurture and welfare of its individual members in their family and community groups. These might be regarded as providing the focus of nursing care and their variety of forms and values as providing many challenges for nurses and other health care workers.
3. Health: the object of all nursing activities whether working for its maintenance or restoration or both. It may be regarded as not only freedom from illness or injury but in a more positive light as an inner conviction of individual and group well-being and a prerequisite for energetic progress towards important achievements.
4. Nursing: the activity of working with, rather than for, individuals and groups in a dedicated relationship in order to maintain or restore health in the broad sense described above. Particularly important might be the idea, not only of the preservation of a life but of the preservation of a good quality of living.
5. Education: a life-long process, whether you are a learner or a teacher, that produces a mature, purposeful, resourceful and efficient person with benevolent views of his fellows and possibly with specialist knowledge, attitudes and skills. Stimulation should be all that is necessary to enhance

motivation and promote a positive approach to learning, while feedback from the supervisor should direct and measure achievement only in so far as this is necessary for the benefit of important third parties.

If this looks remarkably like a brief summary of the whole of the preceding part of this section of the book, you may safely conclude that the philosophy of nursing either has reached the zenith of its vision or that it is desperately in need of your personal philosophical initiative.

The statement of a philosophy of nursing

A last remaining problem is how to turn this mass of recorded and original thought into a statement of a philosophy of nursing which is, at the same time, brief, comprehensive, sensitive, self-explanatory and is preferably expressed with some degree of elegance and memorable, if not exactly exotic, phraseology. The following attempt is submitted for your consideration, not as a model of course, but merely as an illustration of the kind of statement envisaged (Figure 4.2).

This matter of a philosophy has been dealt with at length because it is absolutely fundamental to the curriculum procedure. If you consider these topics seriously and at equal length in a spirit of accord and unity of outlook in your team meetings, the reasons for everything that nurses do and need to know can be made clear; the reasons for desiring certain changes in the ways that nurses behave, for seeking to develop an already attractive and effective personality into one that is recognisably that of a *nurse*, will become apparent. You will have answered the vital question: 'Why is all this necessary?' You will have attained a greater degree of wisdom, as opposed to the lesser achievement of knowledge and the still lower acquisition of information:

> Where is the wisdom we have lost in knowledge?
> Where is the knowledge we have lost in information?
> T. S. Eliot, *The rock*

If nursing, as a unified profession rather than a set of fragmented specialisms, is some day able to negotiate a common philosophy with other important professions in the medical and paramedical fields without negotiating away its independent spirit and collaborative flexibility, it will have placed its intellectual and craft skills at the centre of things and earned itself the degree of respect and affection of the community which has been overshadowed for so long by a certain mawkish sentimentality. It will have gone a long way towards gaining the professional autonomy which should long ago have been granted in return for the dedication and accountability which nurses have exhibited and which society has taken for granted for too long.

Our philosophy of nursing for the general nurse

1. No statement of what nursing is can be static: a philosophy of nursing should be dynamic, growing and developing. It is a basic criterion for the design of a process of professional education and for the subsequent performance of nursing duties.

2. It is held that man:
   - Is of central importance.
   - Has inherent dignity.
   - Is worthy of care, consideration and respect.

   Man is holistic, both greater than, and different from, the sum of his parts: he must normally have autonomy.

3. The nurse's aim is to promote health and self-care to its maximum potential by using a problem-solving approach to:
   - Perform, or help the individual to perform, those tasks which he cannot carry out for himself due to his current state.
   - Co-ordinate and assist the activities of other professional groups and of the family and others concerned in his care.

4. The nurse is an agent of change, operating from a foundation of research-based knowledge, attitudes and skills wherever possible. She acts as:
   - A technician in the performance of clinical functions.
   - A communicator in her professional relationships with people.
   - A carer for those in need of support.
   - An educator for those in need of information.
   - An advocate for those unable to present their own case.

5. A further part of the nurse's duties is the delivery of those aspects of prescribed medical care which are accepted as being part of her function.

6. The nurse should be a participative member of her professional body and is responsible to the profession and to society for:
   - The proper performance of her nursing duties and avoidance of malpractice.
   - The maintenance of her own and other nurses' competences.

   She is personally accountable for the discharge of these responsibilities.

Figure 4.2   Our philosophy of nursing for the general nurse.

References

1. Bevis, Em Olivia, *Curriculum building in nursing: a process* 3rd edn, St Louis, Missouri, Mosby, 1982.
2. United Nations General Assembly, *Universal declaration of human rights*, 1948.
3. Henderson, Virginia, *Basic principles of nursing care* 2nd edn, Geneva, International Council of Nurses, 1969.
4. World Health Organization, Expert Committee on Nursing, *Report of the first session*, Febrary 1950, Geneva, World Health Organization, 1950. (Technical report series no. 24: out of print.)

5. International Council of Nurses, Council of National Representatives, *International code of nursing ethics*, adopted by the Council, Mexico City, May 1973.
6. Royal College of Nursing of the United Kingdom, *Standards of nursing care; a discussion document: interim report of the RCN Working Committee on Standards of Nursing Care (England and Wales)*, London, RCN, 1980.
7. Royal College of Nursing of the United Kingdom, *Towards standards: a discussion document: 2nd report of the RCN Working Committee on Standards of Nursing Care (England and Wales)*, London, RCN, 1981.
8. Royal College of Nursing of the United Kingdom, Society of Psychiatric Nursing Working Group, *Standards of care in psychiatric nursing practice*, London, RCN 1986.
9. United Kingdom Central Council for Nursing, Midwifery and Health Visiting *Code of professional conduct for the nurse, midwife and health visitor* 2nd edn, London, UKCC, November 1984.

Further reading

Chapman, Christine, A philosophy of nursing practice and education *Nursing Times*, 23 February 1978, Vol. 74, No. 8, pp. 303–305.
Ellis, Rosemary, Conceptual issues in nursing *Nursing Outlook*, July/August 1982, Vol. 30, No. 7, pp. 406–410.
Henderson, Virginia, The concept of nursing *Journal of Advanced Nursing*, March 1978, Vol. 3, No. 2, pp. 113–130.
Torres, Gertrude, Stanton, Marjorie, *Curriculum process in nursing: a guide to curriculum development* Englewood Cliffs, NJ, Prentice Hall Inc., 1982.

Chapter 5

Step 2   Choosing a nursing model to refine and reflect the philosophy of nursing

Reminder

- Your choice of a nursing model should confirm the view which you have crystallised in your philosophy of nursing. It gives a firm structure and direction *in nursing terms* to an otherwise abstract statement and refines, clarifies and arranges your ideas ready for implementation both in the education offered by your school or department of nursing and in the nursing activities of the service sector.
- You may decide that a model prepared and published by someone else reflects your views quite adequately. On the other hand, you may wish to produce a model that is partly or completely original.

First, a warning: you will *not* find in this section any profound discussion of the Nursing Model as an entity in its own right. Neither will you find any exposition of the individual nursing models which have reflected approaches to nursing from Florence Nightingale's formulation of what has subsequently been labelled her 'Visionary Model of Nursing' right up to Joyce Fitzpatrick's 'Rhythm Model' and Roper, Logan and Tierney's 'Activities of Living Model, Mark II'. However, you may reasonably hope to emerge from the study of this section with a fairly clear, if rather simplistic, idea of what a nursing model is; how to analyse its contents and evaluate its worth; how to use a model of nursing to help in the construction of your curriculum and enhance its future usefulness; and how to construct your own model from the ideas outlined in your philosophy of nursing if you cannot find a ready-made one that matches your outlook and purpose.

What is a model of nursing and how can it be evaluated?

If you discount the Dinky Toy type of miniature artifact, you have cleared the field for the kind of model with which we have to deal here. We are talking of a relatively simple representation in words and, perhaps, in diagrams too, of a very complex activity: nursing. It has a history extending over many centuries, has changed its essential nature many times and is still changing in response to advances elsewhere as well as those within its own structure. These advances lie mainly in the understanding of society, in the understanding of the working of the individual mind and body, in medical and other scientific and technical knowledge, and in the expectations of clients, their families, communities and governments as well as those of administrators, managers and of the nurses themselves.

Your view of this shifting pattern, its present-day shape and significance and its foreseeable developments has already been summarised and enshrined in your philosophy of nursing in the previous section. This was thought through as an abstraction, almost a vision, and as was suggested, will probably have emerged as a set of unrelated ideas, expressing your personal aspirations and your group's hopes for the future, very much like the randomly-ordered products of a 'brain-storming' session. Nevertheless, as in the case of most brain-storming sessions in any sphere of training or investigation, a number of ideas will have emerged from the discussion with some regularity, prominence and a fair degree of general acceptability as building blocks for the future. In the case of our own philosophy of nursing we identified the particular perseverance and prominence of the ideas of Man, Society, Health, Nursing and Education. On that occasion, by expanding these single words into short, evocative definitions reflecting our true feelings about their true meaning for us, we converted single words into concepts, small packages of pre-fabricated units with special significance.

To take this crystallisation of concepts a step further, a 'model' of nursing is an attempt to gather together your concepts into a still larger and more comprehensive unit of meaning and significance covering the whole of nursing, or at least a substantial part of nursing activity, by systematically linking them together into a longer statement, or by adopting someone else's longer statement. This procedure should turn a random collection of concepts derived from the key words of your philosophy into a logical, well-ordered statement of intention, or programme, directed towards the achievement of that state of affairs in the field of health care which you regard as being desirable for all concerned and as being the particular concern and responsibility of professional nurses. Therefore, to build an effective and useful model in this sense, the concepts must, in the first place, be clearly and concisely expressed and logically linked together in order to present, not so much a vision this time, but rather a practical programme which is realistically attainable, given the resources and conditions which you specify for its attainment. It represents a hardening of your philosophy in the direction of practical nursing applications.

Many nursing models are long and complicated and require a great deal of intensive study and wide understanding of the author's background in order to master their implications. If you wish to study a brief, clear nursing model which is immediately and universally comprehensible, though not formally promulgated as a model, turn to the Declaration on Primary Health Care made by the First International Conference on Primary Health Care Nursing, which met at Alma-Ata in the Kazakhskaya SSR in September 1978. This is a logically ordered, systematic and purposefully linked set of ten concepts aimed at presenting a programme to protect and promote health for all the people of the world by the year 2000.[1]

A conceptual model such as this may often be conveyed, condensed and clarified more effectively in a 'conceptual diagram' or 'conceptual map' and Figure 5.1 represents an attempt to present the Alma-Ata declaration in this way.

Values are implicit in models

Concepts and conceptual models in nursing, more than in any other fields of study and work, are loaded with important values. Your assessment of the value which you attach to every element of nursing mentioned in your philosophy and its model is implicit in the overall goal which you set for the nursing activities of your institution, in the order in which you arrange your priorities among the subordinate aims and in the terms in which you express them in the model. These values may be expressed even more graphically in the conceptual map which you might have made, as you would see by comparing the original Alma-Ata declaration with the conceptual map on page 47.

Raths, Harmin and Simon regard values, in this sense, as 'general guides to behavior' which are started by life-long experience of 'conflicting demands, a weighing and a balancing and, finally, an action that reflects a multitude of forces... what is really valued is reflected in the outcome of life as it is finally lived'. They argue that values show what we tend to do with our limited time and energy: they operate in very complex circumstances and usually involve more than simple extremes of right and wrong, good or bad, true or false.[2]

There are three necessary processes for dealing with values, according to these writers: choosing, cherishing and constantly deploying them in everyday settings. It is usually clear from an individual's expressed aims, attitudes and activities whether or not he or she is motivated by guiding values and what is the general nature or tendency of the values involved. This is, perhaps, more apparent in nursing than in many other activities. Thus, your model should be redolent of your individual or collective values in its exposition and organisation of the concepts of Man, Society, Health,

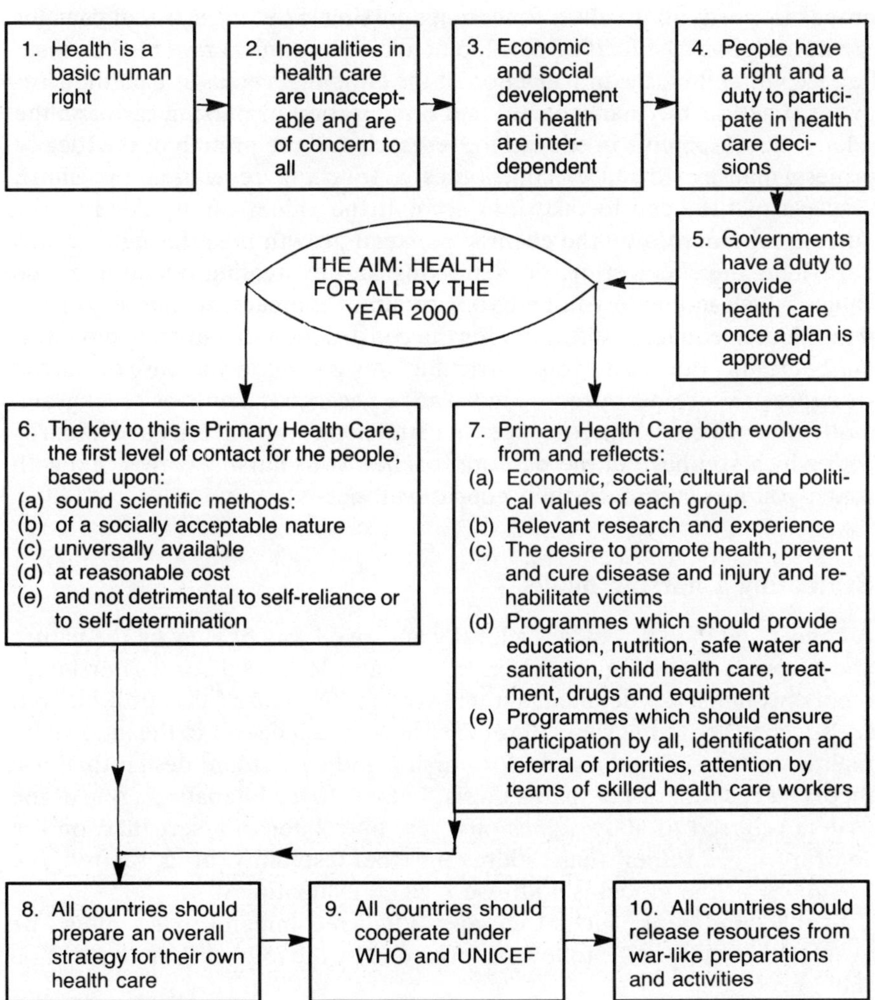

Your own conceptual map may well be less complex than this, but the possibilities are almost infinite.

Figure 5.1 First International Conference on Primary Health Care Nursing, Alma-Ata, September 1978: concept map of the Declaration issued by the conference.

Nursing and Education, or whatever your own choice of concepts might have been. Baroness McFarlane makes the important point that the time is ripe now to reflect upon, and perhaps re-shape and re-organise in a different order of priority, our values concerning nursing. She suggests that changes are necessary in the light of developments in the clinical role of the nurse, her accountability, the introduction of the Nursing Process as a methodology for practice, the management and organisation of nursing care and the related developments in education, research and the growth of the idea of professionalism. She also contributes a touching revelation by Eileen Skellern of the need to take into account the values often added to the nursing relationship by the client's 'personal growth in suffering'.[3]

Perhaps the sheer effort of identifying and expressing openly the true values which motivate you and your group at the current time is in itself more than adequate justification for the construction of a nursing model. It must certainly inject into your curriculum design not only a sense of clarity, structure, order and purpose, but also a necessary depth of feeling and motivation which should convince your students of the sincerity and integrity with which you have in the past approached your nursing career and with which you now approach their educational needs.

Evaluating a nursing model

A conceptual model provides a locally approved way of viewing the nature and purposes of nursing: it is not in any way an adequate theory of nursing. It is not only much less detailed, a framework rather than a full exposition, but is also, contrary to the views of some writers, much nearer to the immediate realities of nursing, education for nursing and curriculum design than is a theory: it is a tool rather than a thesis. In fact, Joyce Fitzpatrick, one of the writers referred to above, goes on a few lines later to assert that, on the contrary, '... rather than addressing the testability of a theory, the *usefulness* of the model is addressed' when evaluating it.[4]

In the same book, Fitzpatrick and Whall recommend that a model be evaluated broadly in the following terms and by the following methods. You should consider:

- Basic considerations such as the definitions of the concepts used to construct the model and the apparent understanding of such basic terms as 'nursing', 'person', 'health' and 'environment'.
- Internal evidence concerning the apparent assumptions of the model and the relative importance, relationships, consistency and adequacy of the main component ideas.
- External evidence concerning the relationships between the model and nursing research, education and practice.

You might wish to reverse the order of the elements in this last item, otherwise it would seem very reasonable to accept this system of evaluating or assessing a model, especially if you follow their recommendations in emphasising rather more insistently the central importance of the concept of the individual client as a holistic, many-sided entity comprising body, mind and soul with social, cultural and personal links and, presumably, a health problem.[4] Nevertheless, with these guidelines, you have a key to the investigation of the nature and overall worth *to you* of any model which you might wish to adopt or adapt.

The applications of a nursing model in nursing and in education for nursing

This short section is offered in the way of a compact summary or recapitulation of what has been already stated or implied in the preceding pages of Step 2, where functions and purposes have been expressed in the course of wider-ranging definitions and discussions of nursing models. The function or purpose of anything is, after all, an essential element in its definition. The functions of a conceptual model which you should seek or construct in order to shape and express your ideas about the intellectually-based craft of nursing are therefore briefly defined as follows:

1. To refine the philosophy which guides your local approach to nursing and to amplify the ideas and their key words to the status of concepts.
2. To clarify and evaluate the values expressed in the concepts and ensure that they are still valid in a changing world and likely to remain valid for the foreseeable future.
3. To set overall up-to-date aims for nursing, especially in the light of the holistic view of the client.
4. To assist in planning improvements in the quality of the care offered to clients by placing all the major concepts of nursing into a systematic and logically-ordered structure and sequence, perhaps in the form of a concept map, so that priorities can be arranged and gaps in the coverage of nursing responsibilities identified and made good.
5. To publicise a firm statement of intention and policy and ensure that it is universally understood and, once approved, pursued by all participants.
6. To serve as the basis of a formal or informal contract negotiated between nurses, doctors, management and, of course, clients, in order to reach agreement on procedures, priorities and protocol in the wider field of health care teamwork.

There are similar applications for a nursing model in the sphere of education for nursing and curriculum design where it is equally, if not more, important to move away from the unimaginative routine teaching of the stereotyped images of even the recent past and, by means of such a model:

■ Produce a blueprint for education which is more than a mere syllabus or list of subjects to be covered and which is, in fact, much more like a detailed and exciting map of a territory that is alive with ideas for action focused upon the clients.

■ Clarify educational values, choices and objectives in the spheres of knowledge, attitudes and skills thus imparting direction and structure to the learning process, keeping it in the nursing, not medical, sphere.

■ Negotiate a contract between the school or department, its students and staff and the service sector, which can explain the purposes and the nature of the education offered and show how it serves the best interests of all three parties and, ultimately, those of the clients.

■ Mark another step in the publicising and implementation of your philosophy of nursing among coming generations of nurses.

■ Assist in the identification and development of areas and topics for research.

For all these reasons, it is crucial to get the philosophy and the explanatory model precisely formulated and expressed in order to ensure that no-one in any sector or at any level of the professions concerned is in doubt about your approach and your intentions. Of equal importance, of course, is the promotion of discussions and contributions in all quarters so as to reach general agreement, acceptance and implementation of a basic model that should ideally be adopted as 'our model' throughout the authority in all nursing situations, even if we are privately aware that the seeds were sown by the school or department of nurse education in the first place.

Choosing an 'off-the-peg' model: two examples

If you are able to assert that, without doubt, one of the many available ready-made models of nursing reflects quite precisely the key-words, concepts, values and attitudes that you have specified in your philosophy and would wish to see re-affirmed, clarified and publicised in your nursing model and throughout the educational process, then you will probably be both very fortunate in having discovered a time-saving short cut in the curriculum design process, and also rather unusual in finding all your views anticipated by another theorist working, in all probability, far away and in a different nursing environment.

Fitzpatrick and Whall offer one of the most comprehensive lists of ready-made nursing models[4] and, in addition as we have noted, they go on to analyse and evaluate each one at considerable length and in accordance with a set pattern of investigation. This feature is most useful since it obviously enables direct comparisons to be made between models competing for your favour. It is clear from even a cursory glance, however, that nearly every model makes a different set of assumptions about Man, Society, Health and Disease, the client, Nursing and Nurse Education.

It is not proposed to investigate any of the seventeen models displayed by Fitzpatrick and Whall, the main objection to such a procedure being its irrelevance to the theme of this book, since it is an essential feature of such a text as this that it should not prescribe for others but encourage them to choose from the widest possible field for their own particular situation. Other objections include the sheer length of the process if one is to avoid making a hasty and ill-considered choice and finally, the fact that all the models, save only that of Florence Nightingale, are of North American origin, coming for the most part from the higher academic levels and intended in many cases as the basis of theories of nursing that are unlikely to surface in this country, especially in our practice. There are exceptions to this stricture which are British in origin, of manageable length and can be related fairly closely to practice. It might be of interest and of some value to sketch briefly the outlines of two models in this category as exemplars of their kind. They are the 'Activities of living' model by Roper, Logan and Tierney[5,6] already in use in this country and the 'Human needs' model by Minshull, Ross and Turner.[7]

The 'Activities of living' model has been based upon the combination of considerations from physiology, psychology and nursing itself, which would appear to anchor it quite firmly in the heart of the client-nurse relationship with some emphasis on the evidence to be gleaned from the observable and often measurable behaviour to be identified with the basic activities of living.

1. These are listed as:
    Maintaining a safe environment; communicating; eating and drinking; eliminating; cleaning and dressing the person; controlling body temperature; moving; working and playing; expressing sexuality; sleeping; dying.
2. These are each liable to be modified by one or more of three approaches to caring by the client and/or the nurse:
    Preventing; comforting; seeking.
    Childhood, pregnancy and old age are singled out as phases of life when activities are such as to require significantly more care and, perhaps, a different kind of care.
3. Five sources of problems are identified:
    Disability; pathological and degenerative tissue changes; accident; infection; and environmental changes involving the physical, psychological and/or social sectors of the client's life.

The continuing assessment of the client's needs is based upon an investigation of this three-dimensional matrix, point by point, and a plan is negotiated with the client in the light of resources and a range of alternative forms of care. The efficacy of the nurse's intervention is judged upon the study of the client's behaviour in each affected sector of his life before, during and after the delivery of care. The nurse's role in caring may be that of an independent practitioner, dependent in so far as cooperation with a doctor's treatment is concerned or interdependent when she operates as part of a team.

The 'Human needs' model of Minshull, Ross and Turner is similarly placed in the immediate area of interaction between the client and the nurse and similarly emphasises the realities of nursing practice so that teaching in the school or department that adopted this model could be seen to be universally understood and translated into practice on the wards if the will to achieve this end is present. It is significant that the 'Human needs' model was created in 1984–5 only because the authors found none of the existing models to meet the criteria for evaluation which they had established; criteria which matched those of Fitzpatrick and Whall quoted above. The most common failing was found to be a still excessive emphasis on the physical aspects of nursing care, so in place of this an adaptation of Maslow's hierarchy of human needs was adopted.[8] The list of needs was accepted virtually as formulated by Maslow in something like the form illustrated in Figure 5.2.

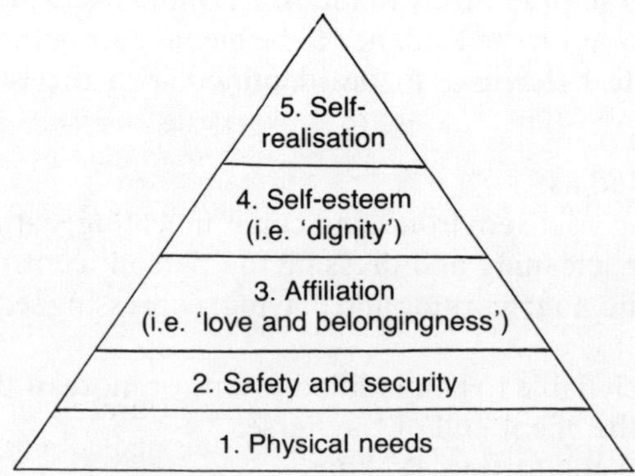

Figure 5.2 Hierarchy of needs.

However, whereas Maslow at first stipulated that each of these needs could be regarded as having been met only when those needs *below* it in the hierarchy or Taxonomy had been satisfied (rather like the pattern of the Taxonomies of educational objectives by Bloom and Krathwohl, if you remember), the authors of this 'Human needs' model regarded them as being independent of each other and as being of equal importance. They held, for example, that the need for affiliation, love and a sense of belong-ingness could very well be satisfied even in the absence of safety and security – possibly even because of their absence – and this is perhaps within the experience of many people: it is possible, though undoubtedly difficult, to preserve or regain self-esteem and dignity in conditions where food, warmth, sleep, security and love are progressively withdrawn. The need for self-realisation may be an exception to this; it is, in any case, a rare and transient area of existence where the nurse cannot intervene effectively and where she can only work at the other four categories of need, leaving the client as free from concern as possible to seek his own self-realisation. Apart from this, the nurse is thought to function along the whole spectrum from total wellness to total illness, incapacity or death and to carry out the processes of assessment, planning, intervention and evaluation as normal.

The fact that this model appears to be very simple and almost self-explanatory need not detract from, and may indeed enhance, its application in all the usual spheres of nursing practice and nursing education. It is, as much as any model can be, a universal model or 'constant' *because* of its simplicity and elegance.

Building your own model

The example of the 'Human needs' model of nursing may have given you some insight into the kind of considerations and thought processes that may go into the decision to build your own model, and into the actual process of construction. These include dissatisfaction with all existing models because they do not feature what you want to express; the identification of one model or some other piece of work, perhaps already familiar to nurses, which could be adapted to your needs; the method of formulating your model, publi-cising it, negotiating modifications in response to suggestions received, finalising it and then beginning the long process of implementing it as a basis for curriculum design and, eventually, for education, clinical practice and, later, research projects.

You will need to define the concepts quite accurately and then ascertain the appropriate order in which they should be placed and the elements of nursing practice to be based on each concept and then define the right kind of language and phraseology to be used to express the ideas properly and to gain the attention and acceptance of your colleagues for this possibly fundamental change in their way of approaching and working through problems in education, nursing, nursing management and research.

You will also need to consider the requirement for constant evaluation, modification and re-evaluation as snags come to light in the early phases of implementation in any one, or all, of these sectors. Further than this it would be imprudent for an outsider to go. This is, after all, your model. You may well complain at this point that you have not been drilled in the writing of nursing models. This is as it should be because each model is a highly individual response to a unique situation. Nevertheless, the brief outlines of the Roper/Logan/Tierney and the Minshull/Ross/Turner models may be helpful to you and in Figure 5.3 a model is reproduced which has been derived from the philosophy to be found in the previous section of this book (see the conceptual map of this model on page 36).

Outline of our Nursing Model for the General Nurse Education Curriculum

1. This Nursing Model has been developed from the 'Philosophy of Nursing' for the express purpose of defining a standpoint from which the nurse's role can be viewed and her work interpreted, planned and executed. It defines the spirit of the venture and therefore the spirit of the curriculum.

2. It is not intended to be a static entity but is expected to be subject to continuing cycles of development and renewal.

3. The approach to the care of the client is conditioned by the view that he is a many-faceted person with physical, moral, spiritual, psychological and social aspects, set in a comprehensive environment. He has his own needs and desires within the natural settings and social conventions of his environment. In the terms of this holistic view of the client, he is seen to have innate worth and dignity and therefore must be shown care, consideration and respect at all times in spite of anything that might indicate a contrary view.

4. The client's health is not merely freedom from illness and injury but is, more positively, his inner conviction of well-being, satisfying integration with his family and community and his eagerness for energetic progress towards important physical and intellectual achievements as well as towards the routine activities of living.

5. Self-care is the client's continuing contribution towards his own health. He should have effective motivation to achieve and maintain self-care in the presence of demands upon and threats to his health and it is the nurse's primary aim to work *with* him, rather than *for* him, to promote and maintain this motivation.

6. Birth, disease, injury, employment, life-style, environmental factors, the establishing of a family, care of elderly relatives, ageing and death represent the range of such demands and threats through the life-cycle. The nurse will assist the client to identify and counter their deleterious effects and to meet his own needs and desires as far as possible, thus fostering the important principle of the client's *autonomy*.

7. The nurse is to be educated to:
   - Promote and supervise the physiological processes of a normal healthy life, of recovery from any of the above hazards to a life of as high a quality as possible or, alternatively, if this should prove impossible or unacceptable, the achievement of a dignified death.
   - Assess the demands being made upon the client's capacity for self-care and establish the reasons for any deficit. These might be lack of knowledge, skill, material resources or motivation and she must then proceed to rectify or compensate for the situation.

- Offer such counselling, advice, support and care as may be necessary and within her competence, involving short-term, intermediate and long-term goals up to and including the client's return to what is, to him, an acceptable, preferably normal, way of life or dignified death.
- Intervene beyond this level of support only if it is deemed necessary to control or reverse a deteriorating situation which, for the time being, the client cannot control or reverse. It must be assumed that he either wishes this to be done for him or is, for the moment, incapable of expressing his wishes in the matter. The aim will be limited to restoring his ability to achieve and maintain self-care and the nurse should be able to justify all aspects of the intervention to those concerned.
- Involve in these activities the client's family and all others immediately concerned by means of acting on their behalf, guiding or educating them and providing physical and psychological care for them as necessary, subject to the wishes of the client.

8. To perform these tasks, the nurse is required to adopt a problem-solving approach within a dedicated relationship which has the effect of placing the client at the centre of the activity. The nurse will have specific responsibilities as a technician, communicator, carer, educator, advocate and deliverer of prescribed medical treatments of many kinds. The execution of these responsibilities will entail the undertaking of basic education to secure sound knowledge, benevolent attitudes and precise skills, the deployment of advanced and, perhaps, specialised, research-based knowledge, attitudes and skills and the search for opportunities to impart these to her professional colleagues who still lack them.

9. The nurse is expected also to be in participating membership of relevant professional associations, to abjure malpractice and to render herself accountable for all that she does in the course of these duties.

Figure 5.3 Outline of our Nursing Model for the General Nurse
Education Curriculum.

It is necessary to point out here that your model, as a development from your abstract philosophy, is not truly completed or confirmed until you have added to it a comprehensive statement as to what your nurses are expected to do in their daily routines and how they are expected to do it. The latter point is dealt with in the next Step when consideration is given to the way in which the idea of the Nursing Process affects curriculum design. The former point is to be explored in Step 4 under the heading of 'The listing of nursing tasks'.

References

1. International Conference on Primary Health Care Nursing, 1st, Alma-Ata, September 1978. Declaration (on primary health care), *Nursing Times*, 16 November 1983, Vol. 79, No. 46, pp. 28–29.
2. Raths, L., Harmin, M., Simon, S. *Values and teaching* Columbus, Ohio, Merrill, 1976.

3. Jean, Baroness McFarlane of Llandaff, Nursing values and nursing action, *Nursing Times*, 29 September 1982, Vol. 78, No. 39, Occasional papers Vol. 78, No. 28, pp. 109–112.
4. Fitzpatrick, Joyce J., Whall, Ann L., *Conceptual models of nursing: analysis and application* Bowie, Maryland, Brady, 1983.
5. Roper, Nancy, Logan, Winifred W, Tierney, Alison J., *Elements of nursing*, 2nd edn, Edinburgh, Churchill Livingstone, 1985.
6. Roper, Nancy, Logan, Winifred, W., Tierney, Alison, J., *Using a model for nursing*, Edinburgh, Churchill Livingstone, 1983.
7. Minshull, Jean, Ross, Kathryn, Turner, Janet, The human needs model of nursing *Journal of Advanced Nursing*, November 1986, Vol. 11, No. 6, pp. 643–649.
8. Maslow, A. H., *Motivation and personality* 2nd edn, London, Harper & Row, 1971.

Further Reading

Aggleton, Peter, Chalmers, Helen, *Nursing models and the nursing process*, London, Macmillan Educational, 1986.

MacNeil, Morag, Models and the curriculum, *Senior Nurse*, June 1987, Vol. 6, No. 6, pp. 22–23.

Ross, Margaret, M., Bourbonnais, Frances, F., Carroll, Gisele, Curricular design and the Betty Neuman Systems Model: a new approach to learning, *International Nursing Review*, May/June 1987, Vol. 34, No. 3, pp. 75–79.

Smith, Lorraine, Models of nursing as the basis for curriculum development: some rationales and implications, *Journal of Advanced Nursing*, March 1982, Vol. 7, No. 2, pp. 117–127.

Smith, Lorraine, Applications of nursing models to a curriculum: some considerations, *Nurse Education Today*, June 1987, Vol. 7, No. 3, pp. 109-115.

Wright, Stephen, G., *Building and using a model of nursing*, London, Arnold, 1986.

Chapter 6

Step 3   Applying the Nursing Process to stabilise the philosophy

Reminder

- A concept of the nursing process must now be clarified and prepared for use in this curriculum design procedure. The major facets of nursing, as you see them, have emerged from your philosophy (Step 1) and have been crystallised and put into their appropriate order and relationships one with another in your model of nursing (Step 2).
- The Nursing Process was quite deliberately omitted from those steps because it does not mark out a theory nor a spirit of nursing activity; it does not define any necessary nursing knowledge, attitudes or skills. It is substantially a tool for examining and organising them, initially in clinical practice but also in education for nursing.
- It is therefore the function of Step 3 to promulgate the Nursing Process for use as a tool to make possible a systematic examination and structuring of each facet of nursing as revealed by the philosophy and model, and of the many 'tasks' of nursing into which your facets will be divided in Step 4, ready for their incorporation into the curriculum.

In a sense therefore, this Step 3 does not carry forward the preparation of the curriculum; it is rather like a short interlude during which you will be able to ensure that you are familiar with both the general outline and the significance of the process and with its function in the succeeding steps of the curriculum design procedure as outlined above and elaborated below. It is appropriate here to reiterate the point which was made at the beginning of Step 2 in relation to the model of nursing; you will not find in this section any lengthy exposition of the Nursing Process and its implications for *nursing*.

Suffice it to say at this stage, for the sake of making our investigation complete and also to ensure that we all start out with the same concept, that this much-debated Nursing Process seems to be a matter of simple commonsense in spite of its uncertain origins and rather turbulent history. It is not a revolution, not even a revelation. It is simply a systematic and effective way of organising the nursing of a client. It recommends that you should identify and assess the normal state, desires, needs and personal and social background of a person who is accepted into your care during a time of crisis for *him*. It is, further, a systematic way of deciding, planning and implementing ways of dealing with his crisis, evaluating their efficacy and progress at suitable interim stages and at the final stage of deciding upon his return to normality or whatever degree of independence is feasible for him. Finally, it is a way of maintaining a 'log-book' or running account of the whole episode.

This is tantamount to treating each client as a small research project and it does serve to focus attention upon the client, rather than focusing on the condition to the virtual exclusion of the client as a person. If such an approach is considered necessary in the case of undertakings in engineering production and repair, in laboratory experiments involving animals, in social work and medicine, among many other similar intellectual crafts, it seems inconceivable that nurses should apparently regard flair, intuition and tradition as constituting by themselves an adequate framework and justification for their own activities. In fact, of course, many nurses have regularly used a nursing process of their own devising or of some local validity, but a greater degree of standardisation is necessary to a proper understanding when clients are now commonly either treated simultaneously by a team of doctors, nurses and paramedical workers or are passed on successively from one to the other as treatment gradually gives way to care and then to rehabilitation. Others in the team or in the chain need to know all that has been already determined and done in the client's case and the Nursing Process lends a pattern and a documentation to ensure that this is clarified.

In nursing it is, of course, a way of doing things or a tool for doing them; it is no substitute for the actual activities of caring or of preventing ill-health or restoring good health and it is in this sense, too, that we must regard it in the context of curriculum design.

In the same way that in nursing the Nursing Process seeks to focus all thought and activity upon the client as an individual rather than upon the routines of the institution and the organisation of the nurse's day, so it is hoped that the influence of the Nursing Process upon education for nursing will similarly focus attention upon the student rather than upon the needs of the school or department or those of the teaching staff. We might usefully investigate how this might be brought about. The influence of the Nursing Process in nursing education may be felt in three ways:

1. It will almost certainly figure as part of the subject content of the courses. Students will be expected to learn about the Nursing Process, what it is and how it is applied in practical nursing. They will, presumably, learn the relevant skills of interviewing, discriminating, decision-making, planning, communicating, teaching and documentation to various degrees of sophistication as suggested by Greaves.[1]
2. The Nursing Process may well provide a model for a similar 'learning-and-teaching process'. In this way, the identification, assessment, and assembly of data, planning a learning strategy, implementing learning and teaching activities, interim evaluation, reflection and readjustment of objectives and methods (which Florence Nightingale interestingly referred to as 'overhauling') and the final testing of the learning accomplished, would be as characteristic of life in the school or department as it is of life in the clinical areas. The one would reinforce the other until the process might become second nature as a way of dealing with problems and activities in all sectors of life. Sylvia Docking has commented on this application: 'It requires teachers to develop divergent thinking skills and to be creative.'[2] No doubt, it would also make the students more free-ranging and more innovative in their thinking and learning.

Both of these aspects of the Nursing Process in relation to the curriculum will be considered in later steps of the design procedure, but now, thirdly, we should, perhaps, consider how:

3. The concepts of the Nursing Process might influence the progress of curriculum design itself. This is our major topic here in Step 3 and it is a matter about which very little has appeared in the literature of education for nursing.

In an earlier chapter — 'Introduction to a closer study of the curriculum design and development procedure: curriculum models', we have already encountered a curriculum model, analogous in many ways to the nursing model. In both cases we have an organised set of ideas or concepts which displays in key-words and a diagram or two, the essential features of a proposed course of action. In both cases we have a natural progression from such a model to the planning and execution of an intellectual activity, in the one case curriculum design and in the other case, clinical nursing. It is feasible that, since in the case of nursing, great benefits in the clarification and organisation of the activity are gained by passing the concepts of the model through the medium of the Nursing Process, so too the activity of designing a curriculum for nurse education might gain in clarity and organisation by having its conceptual model subjected to the same scrutiny, that is, having it passed through the same medium, the provisions of the Nursing Process adapted to serve as a 'curriculum process'.

We may then identify a number of ways in which the curriculum designer might benefit by bearing in mind and applying to the work, the strictures of the assessing, decision-making, planning, implementing and evaluating routine of the Nursing Process from Step 4 onwards.

1. In the first place you could use it to help to ensure that educational and clinical nursing objectives are in alignment, adhering to a common pattern by being derived from the same viewpoint and being focused together by the Nursing Process on to the same problems. In this way, it is hoped that students will find greater identity and coherence between academic teaching in the school or department and practice in the clinical areas in which they may be scheduled to serve.

2. You could also use it to help to ensure that knowledge, attitudes and skills emanating from biological, medical and social sciences and other areas of study peripheral to nursing are similarly reduced to a pattern that is standard within nursing for successful integration into both nursing education and practice.

3. You may employ it as a means of focusing abstract ideas from the philosophy and model of nursing 'forwards' on to the desires and needs of a real or fictitious client at the heart of a case study or simulation, by specifying how these abstract ideas shall be applied to the nursing tasks in the given circumstances.

4. In the opposite direction, proceeding 'backwards' as it were, from clinical practice into education, the Nursing Process can be used to ensure that the finished curriculum design and content reflect the changes in beliefs, attitudes and practices that are making their way slowly through nursing, without the need for the curriculum designer to incorporate the Nursing Process into the philosophy of nursing as expressed at the beginning in the statements of fundamental nursing precepts. It is not a 'key concept' in our sense of the phrase and should not be treated as such but can, nevertheless, be given its rightful place and degree of importance in the procedure and in the outcome of curriculum design.

5. The Nursing Process standpoint and routine can also be used as a valuable influence on the extent to which a fundamentally product-based curriculum with its objectives and prescriptions ensuring control and predictability, economy and quality of its output of educated nurses, can nevertheless be constructed so as to give adequate freedom to the students and indeed, to the teaching staff. Under its aegis they can incorporate opportunities for the identification, assessment, decision-making, planning, learning and self-evaluating processes in education into the basic product curriculum as suggested above by Docking.[2]

6. The Nursing Process can also be incorporated into the curriculum process in order to ensure that what are labelled for convenience, the 'tasks' of

nursing, in the absence or pre-emptive use elsewhere of other suitable terms, are not interpreted as purely psychomotor tasks: things to be done that require only physical skills such as practice and a touch of dexterity. While our curriculum is based upon the analysis of so-called tasks, this term is used very liberally. The analysis in Step 7 uses criteria and factors that centre upon the assessment of the client's needs and desires, upon attitudes towards him, decisions and plans made about and with him, and care implemented and evaluated to bring about his recovery of personal independence. These involve, alongside certain psychomotor skills, a range of quite complex knowledge elements and attitudes evoked by the application of the Nursing Process to the simplest so-called task.

7. In the last analysis, of course, the curriculum designer would be well-advised to apply the ubiquitous principles of the Nursing Process to her own deliberations; the systematisation and the self-discipline induced by their use cannot fail to represent a gain for professional expertise and the quality of the finished product. We can all profit by the 'process'!

References

1. Greaves, Fred, *Nurse education and the curriculum: a curricular model* London, Croom Helm, 1984, especially pp. 22–25 and 78–98.
2. Docking, Sylvia, The challenge of change: the nursing process as a curriculum development, *Senior Nurse*, August 1986, Vol. 5, No. 2, p. 26.

Further reading

Kratz, Charlotte (editor), *The nursing process* London, Baillière Tindall, 1979.
Long, Rosemary, *Systematic nursing care* London, Faber & Faber, 1981.
Marriner, Ann, *The nursing process: a scientific approach to nursing care*, 3rd edn, St Louis, Missouri, Mosby, 1983. A substantial contribution to the study of the Nursing Process, well authenticated by research findings and clinical practice, but American in origin and therefore not altogether appropriate to the British setting.
Nursing Times, The nursing process, London, NT/Macmillan, 1977.
Nursing Times, The nursing process in action, London, NT/Macmillan, 1981.

Chapter 7

Step 4   Listing the tasks of nursing once they have been defined and refined: are they 'professional' tasks?

Reminder

The nature, and by implication, the tasks, of nursing were defined in broad outline by the philosophy (Step 1) and these definitions were refined by the derivation and application of the model of nursing (Step 2). The clarification of the pattern by which nursing tasks were intended to be done, by the application of the Nursing Process in Step 3, has helped to stabilise thes definitions by anchoring them in the realities of everyday nursing practice. It is now time, in Step 4, to make a list of all the activities of this everyday nursing practice, not as might appear at first sight, so as to construct directly from them a 'list of contents to be taught' for the proposed course; the design of a curriculum is a more subtle and demanding matter than that, but at least the listing of tasks is the point at which the educational process begins to look seriously at what the students will have to know and be and do during their first five years or so after qualification and to construct a picture of the kind of people who will be required.

This tends to reinforce the points that have already been made twice: that the term 'task' is used because it is the only term available that does not have other unhelpful meanings, and that it must be interpreted in a broad sense to include not only the acquisition of psychomotor skills, but also the acquisition of knowledge and the nurture and display of suitable attitudes to working situations and relationships. It is almost completely true to say that if a curriculum is to have any structure at all, it must be a structure based upon the aims and nature and, above all, the demands of the practices by which nurses are judged in their everyday activities. This is a soundly educational approach and one which is probably familiar to service staff; one which they can support and with which they can liaise. It does not preclude such vital, if rather imprecise, objectives as caring, counselling or educating, since the list must reflect the key-concepts, priorities and categories of your philosophy and model as interpreted by the Nursing Process.

This may seem to be, at present, an enormously time-consuming effort, one which seems to offer no obvious beginning or end, and worse, one for which we offer little in the way of guidance as to the degree of detail required and the extent of the boundaries to be observed. These fears will become even more pressing as you begin to penetrate past the jungle fringes but this section of the book will attempt to illuminate the problems which, at least, have been foreseen and understood in the preparation of this text.

Suffice it to say that once this listing and the subsequent analysis of the tasks in the list have been completed, you will have a clear, firm and almost permanent foundation of researched and established *fact* upon which to base your curriculum now and throughout all future modifications and renewals for many years to come until the time when nursing has changed almost beyond recognition, if, indeed, that day ever dawns. You will also have incontrovertible evidence of your sources when you are called upon to justify what you have done. Lastly, it is a way of countering the accusation that nurse education is 'too academic' or 'too professional', an accusation to which schools of nursing and, in particular, departments of nursing studies in higher education, may feel rather vulnerable.

Can nursing be a 'profession' if it has 'tasks'?

The first duties of the members of a profession are to know what is meant by a 'profession', to know what kind of profession they belong to, and to know what differentiates it from all other professions. The commonly accepted criteria of a profession are numerous and have combined over a period of many years to create a stereotyped image of the rather over-bearing and remote 'professional person'. In fact, this kind of person is seldom found today except in some of the more antiquated reaches of professional practice. At the other extreme are 'professionals' who are clearly not professional in any real sense: self-styled 'professional' footballers, entertainers, and so on who have been described as sheltering within the 'professionalism of the insecure'.[1] There are also categories of so-called 'para-professionals' who may not aspire to the full status but who are usually sincere and hard-working subordinate colleagues of those who do achieve the full status of professional workers. It is not only interesting but also important to discover where nurses stand in this series of categories.

The question of professionalism in nursing has been explored many times. If nursing can be found to subscribe to a sufficient number and variety of the criteria of a profession to qualify as such, this would cast a very different light not upon what nurses *do*, but upon the circumstances and spirit in which they do it. This view of the circumstances and spirit of nursing tasks would then, of necessity, appear in, and influence the nature of, their educational curricula, removing them finally from the area of training and instruction in which they might otherwise be left. The confirmation of professional status might, perhaps, strengthen the case for the completion of the transfer of nursing education into the higher education sector, but it would most certainly remove the image of the tasks of nursing from the area of simple shop-floor operative skills and show them invested with the intellectual content, strengths and responsibilities referred to in the opening paragraphs above.

This would lead to a curriculum with a very different emphasis, as will be noted later, and offer a complete justification for an overall upgrading of nursing in all its aspects. Professionalism is not just a refuge for the unworldly or a pedestal for the pretentious; it really does have far-reaching consequences which are usually beneficial. The criteria generally accepted as distinguishing professional from non-professional activity are briefly as follows, according to Millerson:[2]

1. It is a full-time occupation with a good deal of single-mindedness in its pursuit.
2. There is a strong feeling of calling or vocation in dealing with vulnerable and often helpless people: financial reward is not always the primary measure of success or failure.
3. The professional supplies the client's *needs* rather than his wants in an important sector of his, the client's, life in complete confidentiality and within the confines of a caring, counselling relationship.
4. There is a marked element of social responsibility in the professional's attitude and this leads to the adoption of a code of conduct or ethics which protects the client against any personal idiosyncrasies or prejudices of the professional worker who otherwise may have a high degree of autonomy. It may also serve, conversely, to protect the professional who abides by such a code from false accusation of malpractice by the client.
5. The professional makes decisions on behalf of his client, after discussing the client's 'instructions' as to the desired outcome. After a purely objective assessment, the professional adviser produces a plan, implements it and evaluates its outcome in consultation with the client.
6. The client may withdraw from the professional's care at any time but is otherwise expected to cooperate in the activity.
7. The professional's skills are based upon theoretical knowledge and practical experience. He claims no expertise outside his own area of competence in his role as a professional adviser.
8. The professional must pass entry qualifications in order to practise, submit himself to specialised education and pass tests of competence in

    order to practise unsupervised.

9. He must keep his knowledge up-to-date, extend it, perhaps into more specialised areas of his profession, and should carry out research in his specialism.

10. His work is licensed and controlled by a professional association which, however, does not undertake the functions of a trade union.

11. He does not advertise his services and since the middle of this century has been much more likely to be in the salaried employ of a large corporation or public authority than to be self-employed in 'private practice'.

12. The former state of affairs by which a professional worker was protected from public opprobrium by virtue of his membership of a self-perpetuating and self-protecting professional association except in extreme cases of malpractice, is no longer as prevalent as it was. It is clear that society is now far more ready to demand that a professional's responsibilities should outweigh any rights which he might have by sole virtue of being a professional, and he must remain accountable to society for his actions in his professional, and to some extent, his private life. He must set and maintain standards.

A distinction has been made by Stenhouse[3] between, on the one hand, the older primary professions of the church, the law and medicine, which minister to the whole person in some matter which vitally affects his whole life, in some way approximating to the nurse's holistic approach, and on the other hand, the secondary professions which minister to only part of a person, for example, his feet or his information needs as in the cases of the chiropodist or the librarian. This can be opposed as an artifical distinction which fails to allow for the extent to which a professional in either category may choose to pursue, or feel justified in pursuing, his trade into the client's life, person or affairs, but it should clarify Millerson's criteria as far as the nurse is concerned and help to place her even more firmly in the area of the primary professions with functions complementary to those of the doctor.

One would hesitate to say that nurses care passionately about professional status; many would probably say that it is of little consequence to them in their daily work and would certainly bring no advantages in its train as long as other people fail to see them in that light. Some others are openly scornful of the idea of professionalism in nursing. However, if for no other reason, it seems desirable to establish a clear stance in this matter because of the considerable difference it makes to the interpretation of nursing tasks.

By importing truly professional considerations of theoretical knowledge, attitudes ranging from disciplined objectivity to the establishment of a mutually caring relationship between nurse and client, and skills, some of which are of a high order of expertise, as in the case of the midwife's role in episiotomy and perineal suturing, the curriculum is changed quite drastically. The curriculum designer is thus fully justified in reflecting the professional tone and requirements appropriate to an intellectual craft profession, which emerge from most attempts to frame a philosophy and a model of nursing. Whether these emerge by tradition or aspiration is of little consequence, they are usually there and nursing inherits or aspires to them by right.

Sue Dickinson[4] asserts that nurses must reiterate and reclaim their right to certain areas of work and certain bodies of knowledge, attitudes and skills which both define their professional expertise and differentiate it from the expertise of others in the same general field, but which have slipped away from their grasp during recent years into the hands of certain categories of auxiliary workers. This might be held to suggest that if auxiliary workers, under whatever name, can carry out nursing care tasks, then nursing care itself is not a 'professional' activity. If, on the other hand, in distancing themselves from the auxiliary workers in pursuit of professional status, nurses move over into more 'cure-oriented, technical tasks', then they are likely to become increasingly regarded as assistants, rather than colleagues, of doctors and surgeons.

The advent of the Nursing Process has helped to restore clinical expertise and bring a new cohesion, as well as efficacy, efficiency and professionalism to the basic tasks of nursing care. It would seem that nurses would be wise to hold on to the life-line of the Nursing Process and await the accolade of professional status, however well-deserved, to come to them rather than to seek it too aggressively or ostentatiously before they have assembled the requisite body of knowledge, attitudes and skills in a more easily recognisable form to justify it.

Why list the tasks of nursing?

The immediate purpose of listing the tasks is to take the process of curriculum design a stage further, from the level of broad strategic thinking to the level of the tactical analysis of day-to-day professional activities that await the newly-qualified nurse during the first five years or so of her professional work within her intellectual craft. The listing is also intended, in part at least, to identify the aims and the roles, functions and activities in nursing that are designed to secure them, especially those which do not change significantly with the passage of time. These, rather than the detailed machinery and methods employed, should be the concern of schools and departments of nursing, underpinning and interpreting the principles of the philosophy and its model.

It is not possible, nor indeed desirable, to specify nursing aims, roles, functions, activities or tasks with exactitude and make detailed descriptions of an absolute precision. Rightly or wrongly, hospitals and similar institutions have grown up as a local response to local needs and nurses and others working with them have therefore been imbued with a degree of insularity, not to say, eccentricity, in the interpretation of their aims and in the performance of their activities, while yet sharing a range of identical or similar tools and techniques.

To pretend otherwise and to act upon that pretence would be to assume inexcusably dictatorial powers and to attempt to 'level down' or to ignore innovation, variety and the beneficial borrowing of ideas across the broad face of nursing in a thousand localities. The third purpose of listing tasks, then, is to strike a careful balance between anarchy and regimentation in the process of defining what nurses are to be educated to do and what kind of persons they should be to do it successfully.

Having identified and listed the tasks, it is intended later to take these tasks – roles, functions and activities – and analyse for each one the combination of knowledge, attitudes and skills by which its achievement by the learner may be assured effectively and economically in ways which will be found not to vary significantly from one institution to another, whether it be school or department, hospital or community base. Then we can arrange for these elements to be incorporated into the curriculum.

Some broad assumptions about the tasks that are chosen for listing

Because of the confirmation of nursing as an intellectual craft profession, albeit an embryonic one, the list of tasks and the qualities and characteristics reasonably to be required of those who perform them will be at once more philosophical, more imbued with principles and more extended into the associated peripheral fields of psychology, sociology and technology than would otherwise be the case. These latter bring into play their own philosophies and principles and offer their own intriguing insights.

Certain broad assumptions about nursing and its tasks stem from this and must be expressed here:

1. Nurses should be skilled in the direct delivery, maintenance and restoration of health rather than in purely routine tasks which have no significant content of caring or skill and which involve no special relationship with a client: in particular, they should not be regarded as technicians or administrators nor used as substitutes for non-nursing staff, but permitted and encouraged to exercise and develop their special attributes as nurses.
2. Qualified entrants to nursing should, therefore, properly be employed as 'intellectual craftsmen' in identifying and analysing problems and in planning and carrying out or supervising the implementation and the evaluation of appropriate solutions within the sphere of nursing.

3. The extent of their functions and activities should be defined as all the legitimate needs and reasonable desires of clients which fall within the remit of the service in that locality.
4. Nursing employers are therefore justified in searching for recruits with reasonably advanced intellectual skills such as the capacities to speedily form appropriate relationships with clients; observe carefully; analyse, synthesise and evaluate data; and visualise, create, validate, implement and evaluate solutions to problems. These capacities are much more relevant to the tasks that are likely to fall to their lot than, for example, knowledge of facts, theories and skills which are not supported by understanding.
5. Nurses will remain for the foreseeable future a reservoir of knowledge, attitudes and skills for general application throughout their particular echelons in the field of health care. From their ranks, a proportion will be regularly recruited for other, more specialised health care professions, such as midwifery. A primary requirement of general nurse education will therefore continue to be the provision of a broadly-based and very thorough health service foundation course so that understanding of the client, his problems and problem-solving methods in nursing will not be ousted from the curriculum by narrower, especially managerial, skills which do not, perhaps, share this understanding and concern. Specialisms of this kind should be grafted on to the nursing root-stock at a later stage, if at all.
6. A unified single-entry-level profession is envisaged, subject only to voluntary movements of personnel as suggested by personal preferences.
7. Similarly, no nurse should ever have her task-based professional education influenced by the possibility that at almost any time, an influx of sub-professional workers, brought by considerations of economic cuts and an emphasis on the public accountability of the service to the Exchequer, would displace her, either into redundancy or into the sphere of lower management where her nursing knowledge might be considered by some to be irrelevant.
8. We are not concerned anywhere in this process with the question of job-analysis which must be distinguished from task-analysis in so far as the former is an attempt to use the data gathered in order to break down a specific job with a view to awarding appropriate pay, status and other benefits to the incumbent. Task-analysis, on the other hand, is a specifically educational procedure aimed at determining the qualities and characteristics which a successful operator should be required to bring to its performance, rather than an investigation into what she could reasonably expect to carry away from it.

Some existing lists of nursing tasks

There have been innumerable attempts to list and organise on paper the tasks of nursing in some kind of system or taxonomy. Although they must not be criticised for not providing instant guides to curriculum design, since in most cases this was not their stated purpose, it may be instructive to examine their outlines to determine whether or not they are approximately what we are looking for. If they do not conform to our needs, we should, perhaps, try to find out why and establish some criteria for the kind of listing that we do need.

Phaneuf's *Nursing Audit Chart Review Schedule*[5] is a basis for such a systematisation in reviewing and evaluating the daily work of nursing staff. In relation to each patient, it calls for the analysis and scoring of some fifty nursing functions under the following main headings:

Application and execution of the physician's legal orders.
Observation of symptoms and reactions.
Supervision of the patient.
Supervision of those participating in care (except the physician).
Reporting and recording.
Application and execution of nursing procedures and techniques.
Promotion of physical and emotional health by direction and teaching.

However, this listing is intended as a framework for the establishment and maintenance of *quality-control standards* in nursing; it is not primarily an educational prescription and lacks the systematic structuring and the foundation of a carefully worked-out philosophy of an ideal list of tasks for curriculum design purposes. Other similar listings occupy the contents pages of virtually every nursing textbook ever written and there are fascinating variations in the manner of their structuring and presentation. Here is the contents list of a major new textbook by Perry and Potter[6], chosen because it is modern, comprehensive and specifically oriented towards nursing skills and techniques — these words, in fact, occur in the title. These are the things that nurses do or in which they assist:

■ Support the patient through the health care system: admission, transfer and discharge; reporting and recording; communication.
■ Safety and comfort.
■ Hygiene: bathing and skin care; decubitus ulcer care; care of the mouth, hair, nails, feet, eyes and eye prostheses (spectacles etc.), ears and ear prostheses (hearing aids, etc.); care of the client's environment.
■ Vital signs and physical assessment: vital signs: temperature, pulse, respiration, blood pressure; physical assessment: skin, hair and scalp; nails; eyes; ears; nose and sinuses; mouth and pharynx; neck; thorax; lungs; heart; arterial and vascular systems; breasts; abdomen; genitalia; rectum; musculoskeletal system; neurological system; mental, emotional, behavioural, intellectual, sensory and motor functions.
■ Oxygenation: oxygen therapy; chest physiotherapy; airway maintenance; emergency life support.

- Medication: oral; topical; parenteral; chemotherapy.
- Fluid balance: intake and output; intravenous fluid therapy; vascular access devices; blood therapy.
- Nutrition: nutritional assessment; oral nutrition; gastric and jejunal feeding; total parenteral nutrition.
- Elimination: urinary elimination; bowel elimination; ostomy care.
- Posture, mobility, ambulation: body alignment and mechanics; transfer and positioning; orthopaedic measures; beds, frames and mattresses.
- Infection control: medical asepsis; surgical asepsis.
- Care of the surgical patient: preoperative care; intra-operative care; postoperative care.
- Dressings and wound care: dressings; binders and bandages; hot and cold therapy; wound care and irrigation.
- Special procedures: specimen collection; assisting with diagnostic procedures

Again, it is important to remember that this is not a prescription for a curriculum. Whatever the actual content of the text itself, this list is, at best, only an aide-memoire in the compilation of a syllabus or course-contents list, essentially based upon *routine procedures* and apparently bearing no evidence of a specifically philosophical appraisal. This is not in any way to denigrate the work itself as a nursing textbook.

D. Middleton's *Nursing – 1*[7] gives the pathophysiology of the various illnesses and the nursing role in caring for patients who have been hospitalised with them: total care refers to the wider aspects and consequences of an illness in social and psychological terms. However, *Nursing – 2*[8] for the second, advanced half of the three-year course is essentially *system- and disease-* centred, offering yet another approach to the listing we seek, but not, perhaps, one that we would wish to adopt for our present purpose because of its particular pre-occupations.

- Genitourinary nursing: overview of the genitourinary system; examinations, investigations and procedures; inflammation of the kidneys; renal calculi; disorders of the tract; social implications of venereal disease; nursing role in venereology; bacterial disorders; fungal disorders; viral disorders; parasitic disorders.

The remaining headings are similarly divided in this general pattern.

- Gynaecology and obstetric training.
- Cardiovascular and thoracic nursing.
- Endocrinology nursing.
- Oncology nursing.
- Care of the traumatised patient.
- The special senses.

- The primary health care team: hospital and community liaison; roles of team members.
- Professional responsibility and ward management: organisation and communication; the ward as a learning environment; using research in ward management; the nurse and the law.

At the other extreme from these two books is the contents list of Roper, Logan and Tierney's *Elements of nursing*, 2nd edition.[9] This, as a listing of the tasks of nursing, reiterates the twelve *activities of living* taken directly from their model of nursing: the acme of simplicity and aptness in its approach to the care of a fellow human being. It is certainly sound enough in its foundations, if not explicit enough in the degree of detail which it offers, because of its origin in its own philosophy and model of nursing.

Nursing and the activities of living
Maintaining a safe environment
Communicating
Breathing
Eating and drinking
Eliminating
Personal cleansing and dressing
Controlling body temperature
Mobilising
Working and playing
Expressing sexuality
Sleeping
Dying

In *Nursing: a creative approach*[10], Ann Faulkner introduces, and in her preface justifies, a different, *client-centred* approach to the delineation of nursing tasks:

- Introduction: overview of the Nursing Process and the holistic approach to nursing; the individual in his normal environment.
- Assessment: the patient on admission; assessment of the patient's needs; the disease process; defining nursing problems.
- Plans for care: care plans; maintaining records.
- Problems and plans for care: towards diagnosis; planning care for patients on a medical ward; planning care for patients on a surgical ward; the elderly patient; the dying patient.
- Evaluation and discharge: measuring outcomes; the patient on discharge.
- Care in the community: life after hospital; community services.
- Conclusion: the changing role of the nurse.

Individualised care can only be given if something is known of the patient as a person. I have attempted to write this textbook from the patient's perspective rather than from a medical systems approach, which may militate against the psychosocial problems of the patient and his relatives. If it could be said that I have used a model for this book, it is a model of nursing as a function which responds to an individual's reactions to deficits in his normal life pattern. This concept is incorporated in the nursing process by assessment of reactions to deficits, which is followed by planning, implementation and evaluation of care as a dynamic, continuous process.   (Preface)

This is much nearer to the ideal which we are seeking in that it is based upon a nursing model and stabilised by the application of the nursing process.

A small document published in an amended form in 1977 by the General Nursing Council for England and Wales is entitled *Training syllabus: Register of nurses: General nursing*.[11] The terminology of its title appears dated and out of keeping with our contemporary views on educational curricula. The approach appears to be, at first glance, similarly proscribed and inflexible as it sets out in broad terms the subjects to be studied but it does have the underlying concept of total patient care albeit divided into three main sections which are required to be learned concurrently throughout training. These are: nursing with first aid; study of the individual; and the nature, cause, prevention and treatment of disease.

The booklet goes on to take a tentative step into the new spirit of education:

When defining the overall aims and the learning objectives for the course it will be important to identify the common core of the curriculum and the expected outcomes of the whole course; the synthesis of nursing knowledge, nursing skills and the body of beliefs and values which support a code of professional practice. The stages of the nursing process, as described by Professor Jean McFarlane, and others, is helpful in a theoretical framework for practice. The use of this method commits all concerned in the various caring/learning situations to a shared approach and a common purpose.

The outline of this 'training syllabus' suggests a further way of approaching the listing of tasks by being, almost literally, a catalogue of such tasks which is presented here in a somewhat abbreviated form:

■ Principles and practice of nursing, including first aid:
  Introduction: history of nursing; organisation of the health service, the Area and the District; personal qualities, beliefs and attitudes of the nurse; code of professional practice; relationships with patients and relatives; place of the nurse in the team; international agencies.
■ General care of the ward unit: e.g. care of linen; storage and custody of drugs, etc.
■ General care of patients and nursing procedures: e.g. reception; discharge; transfer; observing, lifting, feeding patients; giving and receiving reports; care of the dying and bereaved; asceptic technique; peritoneal dialysis, catheterisation, etc.
■ Human behaviour in relation to illness: e.g. family participation in care;

relationship between emotional and physical states; etc.
- Administration and storage of drugs.
- Tests and investigations.
- Nursing care in the operating theatre.
- First aid and treatment in emergencies.
- Preparation for professional responsibility: e.g. communication; personnel policies; appreciation of research; etc.
- Study of man and his environment: e.g. normal growth and development; general structure of the body in relation to function; basic dietary requirements; circulation of the blood; elimination; reproduction; development of mind and personality; family and social relationships; middle and old age; personal responsibilities for health.
- Nature and causes of ill-health, e.g. congenital, nutritional, metabolic dysfunction, infections, etc. Promotion and maintenance of health, e.g. factors and personnel contributing to health maintenance; influence of patient's cultural, home and economic background, etc. Nursing care and treatment of sick people, e.g. observation of the patient in his total environment; assessment of need; making a plan of care; giving care; evaluating the effectiveness/suitability of care, involving for any given disease: knowledge of normal function/structure; causes of the disease; symptoms and signs; reasons for and methods of investigation; normal course and complications; medical treatment; social aspects; convalescence and rehabilitation.
- Practical experiences required: initial care; high and medium dependency care; preparation for self-care following discharge; continuing care of long-term or recurrent illness/disability; care of the dying and bereaved: in acute and long-term medical and surgical wards, in accident and emergency, and in operating theatre; care of mentally ill or mentally handicapped people; community care and home nursing; maternity and neonatal care; child welfare and care of sick children; welfare of elderly people and care of the elderly sick. This should include experience of night duty.

It might reasonably be thought that this document was written by senior nurses working in the field and intent upon planning their own replacements in their own image. This would be understandable, but their work is, on the contrary, closer in form and spirit to what we need than are the textbook contents pages and other lists described above, since unlike them, it was designed especially for the purpose of guiding a course of training rather than a course of reading. It shares with Roper, Logan and Tierney and with Faulkner the advantage of being founded upon a coherent and cohesive philosophy. While not sharing with them the refining and clarifying influence of a related model of nursing, it does nevertheless, enjoy the stabilising effect of the Nursing Process structure.

The GNC document also has a rigid three-fold course structure, based upon the idea of a carefully-chosen common core of knowledge and the ideas of expressed training objectives and the evaluation of the extent to which they are achieved. In so far as these ideas were to be determined locally within each school or department of nursing, the concept of some degree of local autonomy, subject to centralised moderating procedures, augured well for the ensuing process of the local interpretation of this traditional list of 'the subjects to be studied'. It is therefore a useful contribution to our search for a listing of nursing tasks for a basic general nursing curriculum, although, of course, no longer current.

The criteria for listing the tasks of nursing

The criteria which appear to have emerged from this examination of some prominent contenders are, perhaps, best summarised as follows:

1. Any listing of the tasks of nursing ('tasks' being interpreted in its widest meaning) should be purpose-built specifically for curriculum design.
2. It should be firmly rooted in the locally-approved philosophy and model of nursing and should reflect the values which they jointly promote, and preferably even reflect the same key words which are used to describe those values.
3. The list should therefore be more than a mere catalogue of duties, procedures, physiological systems or pathological conditions, however familiar, unambiguous and universally applicable any one of these might be.
4. The list should be so structured and arranged that, like a good taxonomy or classification system, it is easy to pick out the important relationships between topics that are intended by the compilers of the list to be integrated into the teaching and learning that are planned within the terms of the curriculum which is to be based upon it.
5. It should be sufficiently detailed to give stage-by-stage guidance through any course of education based upon it, down to the level of small clusters of two or three lessons and to reflect, upon analysis, all the desirable local variations in the knowledge, attitudes and skills to be offered to the students at each stage. On the other hand, it should not be so detailed as to become an unwieldy or quite unmanageable mass of data which will only serve to discourage and discredit its compilers and the staff who would have to teach to its specifications.

With the above criteria in mind, it was an absorbing exercise to construct a list of nursing tasks (Figure 7.1), extruded, as it were, from our own philosophy (Step 1) and model (Step 2) through the formative and stabilising medium of the Nursing Process (Step 3).

Our list of tasks for the General Nurse Education Curriculum

The expressions 'know', 'value', 'apply' etc. are used here only to clarify the approach to a set of tasks: they are not used as properly formulated 'educational objectives'.

1. General
   1.1 Know and apply skills of learning, library use, researching and reporting.

2. Concepts of mankind
   2.1 Value the inherent worth and dignity of mankind:
   - The central importance of respect and care for the individual.
   - Essentials of clients' rights and client advocacy.
   2.2 Know the nature and significance of individual development in relation to: culture; society; sexuality; education; intrinsic abilities; learned skills; attitudes, norms and values; development of relationships.
   2.3 Know the nature and significance of physical growth, development and aberrations.
   2.4 Know and analyse the nature and significance of the individual's social identity and responses; family; working groups, other groups; social class.
   2.5 Know and analyse the determination of social behaviour:
   - Norms and codes of social behaviour.
   - Norms and codes of social institutions.
   - Aberrations in social behaviour.

3. Concepts of health
   3.1 Know and analyse the factors affecting health: personal; social; cultural; ethnic.
   3.2 Advise on the promotion of health and prevention of illness in oneself and in others.
   3.3 Recognise, and where possible rectify, situations detrimental to health in the general environment; hospital; home; school; workplace.
   3.4 Design, produce and deploy literature, pictorial and other health education resources. Instruct individuals and groups in health education matters.

4. Concepts of nursing theory
   4.1 Know and apply the concepts, functions and presentation of:
   - A theory; a model; a problem-solving strategy; the scientific method, as they may be applied to:
   - the design; production; deployment of systems of nursing care.
   4.2 Know how to determine the existence, nature and extent of individual needs relating to tasks which the client cannot do for himself and which are considered to be the responsibility of:
   - the nurse
   - a multi-disciplinary team which she must co-ordinate.
   4.3 Know how to draw up recommendations for the satisfaction of these needs and to establish goals. (For the techniques of delivering nursing care see under 'Clinical Nursing'.)
   4.4 Know how to measure; validate; modify; re-validate and evaluate in absolute terms the products of the nursing service.

5. Concepts of psychosocial care

  5.1 Use the concepts of general psychology to learn and apply theories of:

- Thinking, learning, remembering, comprehending and presenting ideas and processes of reasoning.
- Perceiving and feeling.
- Motor skills.

  5.2 Learn, practise and apply skills of interpersonal communication in relation to:

- the disciplines of everyday life.
- the crises of the life-span especially: childhood; adolescence and student life; bereavement and grief; marriage and family rearing; personal deprivation and stress; social deprivation and stress; physical ill-health; mental ill-health and psychological problems.

6. Concepts of professionalism

  6.1 Formulate and adhere to the dictates of an informed conscience in relation to the nature and general requirements of professional status.

  6.2 Pursue the acquisition and maintenance of: own and colleagues' competence.

  6.3 Adhere to ethical standards regarding:

- Clarification of issues in nursing.
- Relations with colleagues in professional, administrative and trade union matters.

  6.4 Observe accountability regarding:

- The profession.
- Local and national administration.
- Clients.
- The public.

  6.5 Look to wider perspectives regarding: the nature and extent of involvement with activities outside nursing.

  6.6 Know the likely advantages of formulating and adhering to a wider system of beliefs and values that includes and pervades but transcends the range of nursing activities as defined above. This system itself is not a 'qualification' for nursing, cannot be taught and may, or may not, slowly evolve over a lifetime.

7. Concepts of the biological sciences

  7.1 Know and apply knowledge of:

- The structure; functions; maintenance mechanisms of the body.
- Their development and decay in the course of a lifetime.

  7.2 Know and apply knowledge of the nature, causes and broad outlines of the range of diseases; injuries; other pathological conditions, e.g. starvation, addictions, etc.

  7.3 Know about and relate to the above: pathogenic organisms; toxins; infection; preventive medicine.

  7.4 Know about and relate to the above: the classification of therapeutic drugs; their dosage calculations; modes of delivery; actions; reactions and contraindications; the law relating to their prescription, storage and use.

  7.5 Know about and relate to the above: the respective responsibilities of doctors and surgeons; para-medical workers; other emergency services; nurses.

8. Concepts of clinical nursing

  8.1 Know and adhere to the requirements of the Nursing Process in applying nursing care.

9. The practice of data collection

9.1 Distinguish as sources of data: the client; observations of the client; his family; other medical advisers; other persons.

9.2 Know and compensate for factors which: inhibit; delay; distort essential data.

9.3 Know how to avoid collection of non-essential data.

9.4 Conduct collection of data: conduct interviews; design, distribute and interpret questionnaires; conduct observations in physiological, psychological, social contexts.

9.5 Know and apply local documentation procedures: observe confidentiality; know provisions of the Data Protection Act 1984; know provisions of the local regulations in handling data.

10. The practice of the assessment and evaluation of data

10.1 Conduct assessment of the client's nursing; personal; social requirements.

10.2 Synthesise, collate and interpret data.

10.3 Identify:
- Needs; problems; priorities; level of independence; nursing needs.
- Needs to be delegated to: client; his family and associates; other health professionals.

10.4 Record: data; decisions.

10.5 Distribute information to all concerned.

10.6 Devise objectives and procedures for a nursing care plan in consultation with: the client; his family and associates; other health professionals.
Observing: institutional; legal; ethical constraints;
Using: insight; problem-solving skills.

Sections 1–10 may be regarded as a foundation course in relation to the sections which follow.

11. Practical implementation of nursing care: techniques

11.1 Establish liaison with other health care professionals concerned and coordinate their work if called upon to do so.

11.2 Coordinate the care of the client with the care of other clients.

11.3 Provide a safe environment for nursing care.

11.4 Maintain client's optimum condition: physical; mental; social.

11.5 Deal with problems in: breathing; nutrition; continence; sleep; discomfort/pain; mobility/rehabilitation; infection; dignity/privacy including identity, independence, cleanliness, adherence to values and beliefs; preparation for procedures; carrying out procedures; assisting with medication and self-treatment; helping with emergencies; dealing with death and bereavement.

The learning of the above tasks may be regarded as constituting Level 1 of a Spiral Curriculum (Section 11) of which Section 12 below may be regarded as Level 2, i.e. dealing with the same topics in another 'dimension'.

12. Practical implementation of nursing care: client groups

12.1 Carry out the tasks listed in Section 11 above in a unique or special way with the following client groups: acutely ill; chronically ill; young; elderly; injured; client undergoing surgery; maternity care client; client in the community care sector; mentally ill client; mentally handicapped client.

> **13. Organisation and administration of nursing**
> 13.1 Know and demonstrate the relevance and significance of:
> - The world economic environment; national economic environment; social and ethical thought and events; political influences on health care; social policy in health care; general criteria of health services.
> - The National Health Service; contrasts with other health services; legislative basis of the NHS; DHSS; functions, structure, internal economics of the NHS.
> - Statutory bodies, Royal Colleges, trade unions, etc.
> - Hospital administration.
> - Nursing staff organisation in hospital; ward; community.
> 13.2 Know and demonstrate management skills:
> - Budgeting.
> - Personnel management: leadership; co-operation; occupational health and safety for nurses; disciplinary and complaints procedures; communication in management.
> 13.3 Know and demonstrate skills in basic and continuing education.

Figure 7.1 Our list of tasks for the General Nurse Education curriculum.

The procedure and output of the listing of tasks may be adapted for a typical post-basic course, such as midwifery, in an institution which does not cater for direct entrants but whose students are already registered nurses. Such a listing may omit much of the peripheral study of society, the community and the profession, retaining only such elements as are directly relevant to the particular type of clients or collections of skills involved and may therefore be much more procedure-oriented than would otherwise be acceptable.

In Figure 7.2 is a suggestion for the first phase of a course for student midwives. It has been derived from a philosophy and a model almost identical, as far as possible, to those for the general nursing curriculum which are featured earlier in this book.

> **The tasks of midwifery as a 'post-basic' (i.e. non-direct entry) study**
>
> **1. General**
> 1.1 Revise and apply the skills of learning, library use, researching and reporting in the sphere of educational resources for midwifery.
>
> **2. Concept of mankind**
> 2.1 Value the inherent worth and dignity of mankind, especially the pregnant and post-parturition woman and her offspring.
> 2.2 Revise the nature and significance of the individual's
> - Social development, especially within the family unit.
> - Physical and intellectual development, especially in the stages of intra-uterine and infant development.

3. Concepts of health

   3.1 Revise and analyse the factors affecting health in general.

   3.2 Recognise situations detrimental to health.

   3.3 Understand and value the client as a 'whole person' in a comprehensive environment: an individual with her own aspirations, desires and needs.

   3.4 Accept the basic tenet that in the absence of pre-existent disease or injury or of complications affecting a given pregnancy, the midwife is dealing with a healthy person performing an entirely natural function.

   3.5 Understand that this person should be assisted to achieve motivation, knowledge and skills to attain self-care. The midwife intervenes only when self-care is no longer possible for a period of time; she seeks to restore the client's autonomy.

4. Concepts of midwifery theory

   4.1 Revise the nature and presentation of a problem-solving strategy.

   4.2 Know the basic functions of the midwife's active helping and caring role in assisting the woman to make good any deficits in her capacity for self-care.

   4.3 Know how to evaluate the outcome of the midwife's work i.e. the successful integration of a healthy infant into a valid family unit.

5. Concepts of psychosocial care

   5.1 Revise the application of psychology to caring and communication.

6. Concepts of professionalism

   6.1 Know the law as it applies to midwives.

   6.2 Know and apply the ethics, Code of Conduct, the concept of accountability and the concept of the hazards of malpractice.

   6.3 Know the structure, aims and functions of the midwives' professional association.

7. Concepts of the biological sciences

   7.1 Revise knowledge of the structure, functions and maintenance mechanisms of the body with especial reference to fertility, pregnancy and childbirth.

8. General procedures

   8.1 Documentation: general principles.

   8.2 Drugs: storage, administration and accounting.

9. Antenatal care

   9.1 History taking.

   9.2 General examination:
- Head; neck; breasts; legs; abdomen.
- Blood pressure; weight; urine; midstream specimen of urine; blood test; vaginal swab; antenatal cardiotocography.

   9.3 Parentcraft education.

   9.4 Relaxation exercises.

   9.5 Ultrasound examination.

   9.6 Assessment of the home environment for post-natal transfer to the home.

   9.7 Assessment of client's suitability for home confinement.

10. Labour

   10.1 Admission documentation and history taking.

   10.2 General examination (as above).

10.3 Extended abdominal examination including palpation and auscultation.
10.4 Vaginal examination.
10.5 Urine testing.
10.6 Preparation for labour.
10.7 Care during first stage of labour:
- Specific observations.
- Vaginal examination.
- Urine testing.
- Alimentation, with action to avoid or correct dehydration.
- Elimination.
- Pain relief, including relaxation, use of drugs.
- Demonstration and use of the positions of labour.
10.8 Care during second stage of labour:
- Specific observations.
- Episiotomy.
- Delivery of baby.
- Care of baby at birth including identification; initial examination.
10.9 Care during third stage of labour:
- Conservative management.
- Active management.
- Examination of the genital tract.
- Examination of placenta and membranes.
- Perineal repair; suturing.
- Notification.

11. Special considerations appertaining to home confinement
11.1 Care during labour (as above).
11.2 Use of drugs, including acquisition; storage; disposal.
11.3 Disposal of placenta.
11.4 Care of baby at birth (as above).
11.5 Summoning medical aid.

12. The new-born baby
12.1 Immediate care after delivery.
12.2 Extended examination.
12.3 Initiation of breast feeding.
12.4 Initiation of artificial feeding.
12.5 Observation of the baby: labels; colour; respiration; activity; tone/cry; skin; head; eyes; mouth; cord; urine; stools; temperature.

13. The puerperium
13.1 Immediate care.
13.2 Continuation of breast feeding.
13.3 Continuation of artificial feeding.
13.4 Transfer to ward, including observation of lochia; bladder; uterus.
13.5 Care on the postnatal ward:
- General examination: temperature; pulse; blood pressure; urine output; bowel function; uterus; lochia; perineum; legs.
- Observation and necessary action in mother–baby interaction.
- Sleep/rest.

- Exercises.
- Blood tests.
- Use of drugs.
- Postnatal ultrasound.

14. Transfer home
   14.1 Discharge visit.
   14.2 Consideration of environmental needs: mother–baby interaction; warmth; security; safety; hygiene; prevention of infection; caring for the baby's skin, eyes and orifices; handing over to Community Nurse.

Note: Each of these headings would normally be expanded by a number of standard sub-headings to indicate such activities as 'communication with patient', 'interpretation, evaluation and documentation of findings', etc.

Figure 7.2 The tasks of midwifery as a 'post-basic' (i.e. non-direct entry) study.

Note that the tasks in each list have been numbered for ease of reference during later stages of the curriculum design process. In each case the number of headings produced is about two hundred and fifty or three hundred, rather more in the case of the procedure-based post-basic midwifery course when it is expanded by the sub-headings referred to at the end of the tabulation. This appears to be a manageable number of tasks and has been observed to be the average outcome of various curriculum design operations in a number of different professional courses.

Incidentally, there is no intention that these lists should be regarded as being exemplars of any special merit — they are merely offered as an indication of what a list of tasks might look like on completion.

Before we proceed to utilise these lists in the next stage of the curriculum design proper, it might be thought appropriate to take the opportunity in Step 5 to look more closely at the nature and philosophy of *education for nursing* in order to determine what kind of philosophy is best fitted to support and suffuse our version, just as in Step 1 we carried out a parallel investigation into the nature and philosophy of nursing itself.

References

1. MacKenzie, W. J. M., The ingredients of professionalism (part of the Report of the Gulbenkian Educational Discussion on Higher Education for the Professions) 1965, *Universities Quarterly*, March 1966, Vol. 20, No. 2, pp. 147–208.
2. Millerson, Geoffrey, *The qualifying associations: a study in professionalisation*, London, Routledge & Kegan Paul, 1964.

3. Stenhouse, Lawrence, Research in librarianship: an address to the Library Association's Library & Information Research Group at the University of Leeds, November 1972, unpublished.
4. Dickinson, Sue, The nursing process and the professional status of nursing, *Nursing Times*, 2 June 1982, Vol. 78, No. 22; Occasional paper Vol. 78, No. 16, pp. 61–64.
5. Phaneuf, M., *The nursing audit*, New York, Appleton-Century-Crofts, 1976.
6. Perry, Anne G., Potter, Patricia A., *Clinical nursing skills and techniques: basic, intermediate and advanced*, St Louis, Missouri, Mosby, 1986.
7. Middleton, D., *Nursing – 1*, Oxford, Blackwell Scientific, 1983.
8. Middleton, D., *Nursing – 2*, Oxford, Blackwell Scientific, 1986.
9. Roper, Nancy, Logan, Winifred, W., Tierney, Alison, J., *Elements of nursing*, 2nd edn, Edinburgh, Churchill Livingstone, 1985.
10. Faulkner, Ann, *Nursing: a creative approach*, London, Baillière Tindall, 1985.
11. General Nursing Council for England and Wales, *Training syllabus: Register of nurses: General nursing*, London. GNC, amended edn 1977.

Further reading

Chapman, Christine M., Concepts of professionalism *Journal of Advanced Nursing*, 1977, Vol. 2, No. 1, pp. 51–55.
Hardy, Leslie, Engel, Joyce, The search for professionalism *Nursing Times*, 15 April 1987, Vol. 83, No. 15, pp. 37–39. (The nursing process might be a route to professionalism but its boundaries are too narrow and it encourages conservatism.)

Chapter 8

Step 5   Defining the nature of education for nursing: another 'philosophy'

Reminder

This is an opportunity to step aside for a short interval from the curriculum design process and to consider what kind of education we wish to provide for our nurse-learners and, even more important, what kind of education would best match their needs. Since we have so little information about their expressed desires in the matter, it is difficult to take these into consideration. Students themselves have written virtually nothing about their views on the broad outlines of nurse education and we have only our own impressions of their reactions for guidance.

All we can say for certain is that they appear to respond better to education than to training or instruction and that consequently we should, perhaps, offer them a broader, character-shaping education *for* nursing rather than a narrow grounding, however thorough, in the inward-looking routines *of* nursing. One may further suggest that educational methods which involve the student in searching, discovering and creating by using knowledge and experience, appear to produce happier and more competent nurses with wider intellectual horizons than do conventional methods of training or instruction.

One definition of education for nursing could be that it is a process which, when effective, increases the competence of students and enables them to use their benevolence for the promotion of human health and for the care of people who are ill. There are at least three strands interwoven in this process. The first strand could be the nature of students. The second strand could be the nature of those who shape the process of education. The third strand could be the nature of the knowledge of facts and skills thought to be necessary for the promotion of human health and the care of people who are ill. If these three strands are now analysed and then integrated the result could be suggestions for the nature of education for nursing.

In the definition of education for nursing it was assumed that students who elected to become nurses, who were selected and who stayed the course, would be benevolent. Therefore, if the selection process were effective in detecting benevolence, the chosen students would be well-motivated and have an attitude disposed to promote human health and to care for people who are ill. Such an attitude would suggest the capacity for habitual, spontaneous and genuine acts of kindness. If the process of education were to enable such a capacity to become an ability, then each student could make her unique acts of kindness effective for the promotion of human health and for the care of people who are ill.

It seems that students start with a common attitude of benevolence, and a common need for knowledge of facts and skills. Despite this similarity, it would be a shock for any one student to meet her double and so it can be assumed that each student is unique. Students come from differing cultural backgrounds and, although they have one attitude in common, they might have other differing attitudes derived from differing beliefs, such as beliefs about the sources of morality. Other differing attitudes might be derived from customs such as child-rearing methods or behaviour towards older members of a society. Within these various complexes of ideas and activities, each student seems to have a unique psychological status so that even within their common attitude they probably differ in the extent of their commitment to their vocation and in their ideas about its realities. They probably differ, too, within their common need. Some students will start with a more extensive knowledge of health and with more of the skills of caring than others. Also, people generally have differing capacities and because of this and of differing previous educational experiences, they have differing abilities. Thus, some will be more numerate than others and some will be more familiar with, and skilled in the use of, the language by which knowledge is specified and skills are described. Further, during learning students will react differently to the responsibility of searching for knowledge and to the responsibility of cooperating with others for the care of people who are ill.

Then, during the process of caring, they will differ in the management of their own reactions, such as reactions to the stress of physical fatigue and to the witnessing of human suffering. In order to increase the competence of students who are accepting such challenges, great skill and empathy are required from those who shape the process of education for nursing. This shaping ranges from global influences on education to the influence of the nature of an individual student.

Global influences on education for nursing emerge from the ideas of educators and nurses and from the dissemination of these ideas by the mass media of communication. Some ideas are tested by research and are made known by the circulation of research findings in various publications such as journals and abstracts. Such influences spread when opportunities are available for geographical mobility for tutors and nurses. The quantity and quality of these facilities are affected by the ethos of the age with regard to education and health. Also, societies differ in the extent to which ideas are realised. The extent and the quality of resources within a society are affected by the economic condition of that society and also by the position in its hierarchy of values of 'education', of 'the promotion of human health' and of 'the care of people who are ill'. A society's values can be reflected in its laws and in its customs, and so bodies such as law-makers and, in some societies, religious orders, influence education for nursing. It is within this wide-ranging framework that educators shape the process of education for nursing.

The process is shaped by the qualities and educational standards which are used by interviewing, examining and moderating bodies as criteria for the selection and, later, for the assessment of students. Then there is the influence of those who devise curriculum form and content and select materials, and of those who appoint and organise the deployment of educators. In all of these, as in other matters, professional nursing bodies can be influential and prepare the way for those selected educators to use their knowledge of facts and their skills to aid students to increase their competence.

The quality of education is influenced by the care with which a tutor presents facts, criticises ideas and demonstrates skills, including the skills of caring both for students and for those who are ill. A tutor who cares for a student as an individual, whole person is demonstrating this care. The skill of listening in order to ascertain the real needs of a student, the skills of sustaining a downcast student and of appreciating another student's joys, the skill of precision in record-keeping and in the strict observance of confidentiality are examples of behaviour patterns which are of use to a student. When the student participates with a tutor in the care of those who are ill, the tutor demonstrates precision in techniques and at the same time can demonstrate the value of each individual person as being precious. This is loving care being witnessed and shared by a student. When a vocation is concerned with caring for people there is confirmation of the existence of love. Some give love without searching for the source of it; others search and some of these acknowledge that there is something beyond human understanding which touches people in the form of human love. Sometimes those who share this acknowledgement meet to uphold their faith. Faith usually entails a commitment to a particular behaviour pattern. In some cases it determines what is thought to be right in human relationships and so gives moral guidance.

Students face grave moral issues, such as that of determining their own attitude to the human foetus. Moral decisions are also required when caring for people who are ill and who, for example, ask questions about their own illness. A clarification of the concepts of moral discourse and readings and discussions about moral dilemmas might aid all students to make moral decisions. Stress sometimes results from moral dilemmas, physical fatigue, close proximity to human suffering or from overwork. In order to reduce stress, students need facilities for the promotion of their own health, facilities for aesthetic experiences and time to be shared with friends. Aesthetic experiences and friendship can reduce stress and enable students to radiate joy. If the process were shaped with a regard for these matters then each student would be educated as an individual and also as a whole person with needs in addition to the need for knowledge and skills.

What is the nature of the knowledge of facts and skills which are thought to be necessary for the promotion of human health and for the care of people who become ill? Such knowledge is affected by the individual differences in people. Although people can be categorised to some extent, for example into males and females, the people we meet seem to differ in some other ways so that what seems to be true about some people is not necessarily true about others. A further obstacle to knowing about people is that observations about particular persons cannot be represented as a precise description of what is directly observable. For example, it is impossible to give a perfect description of a friend's face. Consider also how difficult it is to represent what is physical but not directly observable, such as the same friend's brain. However, these are simple matters when contrasted with the difficulties of representing the sensations and the thoughts of a friend or the mind of a stranger.

The acknowledgement that there are difficulties in knowing about people suggests that there is a need for forethought, care and candour on the part of the educator in helping students to know how to promote human health and how to care for people who are ill. Also, students who want to be of service to humanity in this way deserve a regard for their integrity and this suggests that the educator's forethought could include an assessment of the degrees of credibility in what students are expected to know. So what can be said that can be known to correspond with the state of things? Some knowledge can be accepted as true. This comes from direct evidence to the senses, such as seeing that something is as it is. Sometimes there are instruments, such as the microscope, which make an observation possible and so this knowledge can be accepted as true. Other instruments quantify evidence, and credibility depends upon the validity and the reliability of the instrument and also upon the observer's understanding of quantification. So far, this kind of knowledge can be accepted as true by students. However, when direct observations provide insufficient evidence, inferences are used.

Inferences are likely to be credible if the evidence used is true and if the argument is valid. Further, when time reveals to the student the truth of an inference, then the inference becomes more credible and, generally, credibility increases with repetition of the verification witnessed by the student. Students lack the time to verify everything and so they watch others making observations, using instruments and making inferences. Sometimes students witness the results of such inferences, but at other times their knowledge is acquired at second-hand. Examples of ways of coping when there is a lack of time to verify everything visually include the use of television programmes, videotapes, films, slides, models, photographs and illustrations. Credibility here will depend upon trust by the students in the makers and selectors of the materials. Another category of aids includes books, periodicals, radio programmes and sound tapes. Here credibility depends upon the students' understanding of language and, again, on trust by the students in the authors, makers and selectors of these aids.

Sometimes the information presents research findings. In order for a student to decide whether or not to accept these findings, a knowledge of experimental design would be necessary. If this were not possible, then credibility would depend upon trust by the students in research workers or trust in the competence of a tutor to evaluate documented research on their behalf. When visiting lecturers present their research methodology and their findings and time is allocated afterwards, questions can be asked by tutors and students in order to clarify the evidence and to test credibility. Questioning and subsequent clarification of evidence which tests credibility is one of the advantages of the lecture method if time is allocated for this purpose. A similar advantage emerges from group discussion following the presentation of a topic and also from the one-to-one meetings of a student with a tutor.

When a tutor enables a student to acquire knowledge, the tutor is demonstrating skills similar to those which the student requires for the promotion of human health by means of health education. One such skill is that of searching for new information including the information required to use the beneficial products of technological change or to cope with new hazards to health.

Other skills are necessary in the care of people who are ill. For these skills a student requires both a knowledge of the procedures and the ability to perform tasks with precision. Some are well-tried procedures which demand meticulous care along an established prescribed route, sometimes alone and sometimes in cooperation with others. A tutor who uses such care in procedures in the presence of a student is presenting the reality of what a student hopes to become. Probably someone who has selected nursing as a career will be well motivated to acquire such skills in the presence of a skilled practitioner of nursing. Tried procedures are not available in all circumstances and so, in addition to the skill of caring along an established prescribed route, the skill of assessing a particular situation and then of designing a procedure or care plan under the supervision of an experienced tutor might prepare a student for the devising of procedures for innovation, and sometimes for improvisation, in the future. These innovative procedures, sometimes carried out by the individual and sometimes in cooperation with, or in liaison with, others would be necessary at times of unexpected emergencies in any part of the world at any future time. Such emergencies might be the result of geophysical events such as earthquakes, volcanic eruptions and floods or they might be due to organic causes, such as widespread infections. Other emergencies could arise, as in warfare and other forms of violence, and also as a result of the introduction of technological changes in the environment, such as the introduction of a different form of fuel.

Innovative procedures need not be limited to use in emergency situations. They could be devised as an improvement on existing procedures. Also, innovation would be necessary in order to utilise ingenuity in technological advances for the promotion of human health and the care of people who are ill. So far the skills have been those of either established or specially devised procedures. Such skills are fairly clearly defined. Generally, however, the skills are applied to people and the skills of knowing how to behave with people are less clearly defined. One reason for this lack of clarity is that different people might react differently in a similar situation such as in their feelings of vulnerability when carrying out private acts in a more public setting than is usual.

A second reason for the lack of clarity lies in the difficulty of the problems to which skills are applied. Some practical difficulties might be easily overcome by liaison with specialists. An example would be that a skilled translator could overcome the problems of knowing how to behave with someone who was ill and who could not understand the language and the culture of their present environment. Even here there could be problems; for example, if the translator were not sufficiently skilled he could misinform the carers. Then, in addition to practical problems, a carer is confronted by life's more profound problems. These include, for example, the problem of knowing how to behave with a child whose parents have died; with a young person who will be dependent upon others; with a family man or woman whose illness separates them from their children; with an elderly person whose illness separates him or her from an ageing, frail partner; when witnessing another's pain or when listening to someone's reactions to the prospect of death. The skills of caring in these circumstances would be practised by experienced nurses, sometimes in a one-to-one relationship and in these cases the presence of a student might interfere with the exercise of the skill. Also, a student might err unwittingly and cause suffering to someone already overburdened with difficulties. Discussion with tutors and role-play, followed by discussion with appropriately experienced practitioners would prevent the student from making errors such as that of raising false hopes. Then published ideas, further discussion and reflection would begin the building of a skill on the foundation of an attitude of benevolence.

We have considered the definition of education for nursing, the nature of students, the nature of those who shape the process of education and the nature of the knowledge of the facts and skills which are thought to be necessary for the promotion of human health and for the care of those who are ill and this has resulted in the following suggestions for the nature of education for nursing:

1. Education is a process which respects every individual student's uniqueness and at the same time helps them to fit themselves for: activities within an established system where they can benefit from the knowledge and experience of others; innovative activities at some future time either as an adaptation to circumstances at present unknown or in order to improve on an existing system.
2. Each student is a whole person, so the educator could: sustain their physical vitality for their strenuous vocation by aiding them to gain information for self-care and by providing facilities for a variety of enjoyable leisure activities; provide for their need to acquire a knowledge of facts and skills for their vocation and enable them to verify evidence so that they come to know authentic facts and skills; educate partly by training in the presence of experienced practitioners and partly by providing opportunities for searching, discovering and creating by the use of factual knowledge and of experiences; provide opportunities for students to witness and participate in loving care in order to foster their benevolence; acknowledge that nurses face grave moral issues and provide facilities for the discussion of these, including a clarification of the concepts of moral discourse.

The three 'strands' listed at the beginning of this Step, which may be briefly designated as the students, the tutors and the educational process, represent two factions and an arena. The scene is set for the possible development of conflicts which can only be controlled by the utmost goodwill on the part of both factions and the mutual negotiation, rather than unilateral imposition, of many aspects of the educational process. One should, perhaps, consider also such factors as the present dual role of both students and tutors, divided between the educational and clinical spheres; the impact of third and fourth parties, the clinical practice personnel and the clients; the contrasts between young adults and older adults in all the groups involved; and the stresses of the world of caring in an age of severely restricted resources, especially as regards limitations of time and funds.

Key words already used in the course of the last few pages may serve to highlight potential dilemmas in the situation and suggest further sources of conflict: 'procedure' versus 'innovation' and 'integrity' versus 'reactions to human suffering', for example. Other key words used suggest possible paths to reconciliation: it is the function of the educator and the tutor to exercise 'candour', 'care' and 'forethought' in a diplomatic and, above all, compassionate manner in all aspects of their work. In the last analysis, they have the responsibility to specify the range of possible conditions to be negotiated, while the students usually have little option but to react to these specifications. Equilibrium, when finally achieved, is the measure of a mutually satisfying relationship.

Chapter 9

Step 6   Defining the categories of knowledge, attitudes and skills available in an educational process

---

Reminder

We have not yet arrived at the stage of injecting subject content into the curriculum because we must first consider ways of ensuring that the students who are to receive the knowledge of subject content are concurrently transformed into the particular kind of people who are best fitted to use it in the practice of nursing. Subject knowledge by itself will not do this. Once transformed, they are professionals in the special sense that they are equipped, not only with routines, but also with understanding; they are resourceful and they will become adaptable and innovative in due course. The curriculum must be shaped to promote what is to a large extent a special outlook, rather than merely a special package of subject content.

The 'Table of Learning', with its list of various kinds and levels of knowledge, attitudes and skills and the means of attaining them, enables the educator, through the medium of the curriculum, to choose carefully an appropriate selection of knowledge, attitudes and skills from column 1 of the table, plan their development and emergence in the learning process, enhance their effect, and cause them to merge and cumulate towards the production of the desired kind of nurse. This can be done by providing her, throughout her time as a student, with relevant experiences in knowledge, attitudes and skills, indicated by column 2 of the table as tending to produce the desired achievements listed in column 1.

Subject matter becomes important later as a filling for the framework of learning which produces these changes. Of course, at this later stage, subject matter is important in its own right in that it directs the nurse as to what to do, while at the same time, it gradually changes her so that she can do it in a more truly 'professional' and 'nurse-like' manner.

The purpose of this Step 6 is to prepare ourselves for the activity described above and dealt with somewhat more extensively in Step 7, by now examining the nature and significance for us of knowledge, attitudes and skills, so as to be in a better position to make recommendations about their selection and deployment in the special case of education for nursing.

The target for the educational process

In so far as the acquisition of expertise may be interpreted as the acquisition of experience, that is, the cumulation of knowledge, attitudes and skills over a substantial period of time, we may find it useful to describe the successive stages by which a desirable level of performance is achieved. This might enable us to gain some insight into the way in which these qualities affect the individual learner's output of work and way of life and thus give us some idea of a target for the curriculum which we are designing to deliver those qualities – that is, a nurse with the potential for expertise.

Patricia Benner[1] has analysed and described the stages of the average nurse's career. The novice/beginner lacks experience and so she tries to follow the rules implicitly in her daily work, does not exceed them and certainly does not bend them. She may lack some elements of understanding and be sufficiently unaware of principles as to consider it too great a risk to use discretion in even the simplest and most common decisions about, say, family visiting patterns for her hospitalised patient. The practising of basic skills occupies most of her thoughts. There comes a time, however, when the nurse reaches a more advanced stage of the beginner's saga; though still preferring the security of rules, she becomes rather more flexible and is prepared to consider the possibility of following somewhat less rigid guidelines which give her occasional opportunities to use an element of discretion in timing and arranging her work in contact with the client for the latter's benefit. She is able, and rather more willing than before, to discuss these matters and enjoy a concession while equally accepting that she must conform to the relevant rules when given sound reasons for doing so. Her problem is not so much one of seeing all or most of the aspects of a situation but in deciding upon priorities among them. The perfecting of basic skills becomes a distinct possibility but the day is still a series of uncoordinated tasks, each of which comes as something of a challenge.

As we have seen already, *competence*, although a worthy aim, is far from being the end of the story. It comes to most of us after the first two or three years of work. Efficiency and generally sound organisation of work develop, the day is planned as a whole rather than as a series of uncoordinated tasks and, on an even longer time-scale, some forward planning is done well ahead of schedule and a career is envisaged and launched. Confidence and the ability to cope begin to emerge, although rules and guide-lines are still consciously and conscientiously followed.

The *proficient* nurse appears to move beyond this stage. Procedures have been perfected; priorities can be decided on the basis of experience; situations can be analysed at a glance and activities planned on the basis of reasoned discussion. *Expertise* may be described as smooth and speedy, as well as efficient, working, together with the intuitive summing up of normal situations, with the processes of conscious analysis and decision being deployed only in the face of the unusual. This is the result of careful preparation in terms of curriculum design, content and teaching, with the addition of self-critical monitoring of experiences and continuous learning as a way of life. Herein lies the importance of selecting the right blend of knowledge, attitudes and skills throughout the curriculum design process and adapting them not only to the needs of a particular school or department of nursing, but, in the last analysis, even to the needs of an individual student. This is the message of Step 6 of the procedure.

With regard to these three categories of learning, the Nursing Process Evaluation Working Group[2] has recently reported on the following lines, assuming that the Nursing Process be implemented in schools and in the service sectors associated with them:

> This means that the nurse required enough *knowledge* to assess, prescribe, carry out and evaluate the care she gives. In turn, this implies knowledge of normal human functioning... coupled with the knowledge of how to apply this in nursing exigencies, for example, the management of pain... Additionally, a knowledge of fundamental human relations... is essential. Awareness of research findings and the ability to relate them to all these areas is important. Side by side with such aspects stands the necessity for a considerable knowledge of medical interventions and their likely consequence for nursing care.
>
> The use of the nursing process calls for a fundamental change in *attitudes* between patient and nurse. The patient becomes a partner in care, the nurse becomes accountable ... There is a consequent change of relationships between the responsible nurse and the nurse managers.
>
> To practise the nursing process successfully the nurse requires a wide range of *skills*. Some of these skills are particularly relevant although not exclusive to any one stage...

It is particularly significant that most of the skills listed are interpersonal skills such as communication and intellectual skills such as measurement, analysis and judgement. Psychomotor skills are listed as a category under that heading but are not differentiated in what is admittedly a short and selective list of skills. The present analysis in this Step will have to take account of this distinction and of the range of skills that are purely manual.

Here, then, is a confirmation of the validity and relevance of the three-fold division of nursing tasks, although too much should not be made of the distinctions between them which are, to some extent, a matter of convenience for the curriculum designer. It is now appropriate to look at the nature of each of these categories in greater detail so that we can assess more accurately just what mix we need to achieve the level of competence, if not proficiency or expertise, in the tasks briefly outlined under the same headings by the Nursing Process Evaluation Working Group and expanded in the list of nursing tasks already prepared in Step 4.

The nature of knowledge

Before attempting to describe the nature of knowledge and fixing its limits, it may be thought important to clarify some of the ideas involved so that we can arrive at some agreement about their meaning and significance.

'Knowing' is an idea of considerable interest. To 'know' is something that is not covered by the natural laws of the universe. It is an activity or state which is within the mind and there is no evidence for the existence of the mind as a natural object alongside the liver and lungs. Nevertheless, it is a powerful force, a set of processes, a first-hand experience, an awareness which is apparently known to, and reported by, every person who is not severely physically or mentally disabled. It may be carried on in part of the brain but beyond that we find it difficult to account for the concept of 'me-ness': the idea that 'I' am a distinct and different package of existence from everyone and everything else. It implies acceptance of what is observed, belief in what is accepted, the appreciation of the truth about what is observed and believed in, and the capacity to use what is held to be true for the purposes of surviving and enjoying and enhancing the future into which we hope to survive.

'Knowledge' is the individual or public record of the truth as a whole or as it is seen in a particular place at a particular time; as such, it appears to be a formidable entity: boundless, shifting and uncontrollable. Some thinkers maintain that the reality of knowledge lies only in what we can see and touch; others, the sceptics among us, go to the other extreme and assert that since we cannot penetrate the screen of illusion presented by what we see and touch, we can never know the truth. A common-sense view might suggest that the people, things, events and places that we can see and touch are real enough for all practical purposes although they probably, or possibly, do not represent the whole of reality, and what the rest of reality comprises is often literally a matter of faith. One way of seeking to investigate and control knowledge is to categorise the things, people, places and events which it observes, as a start towards making an inventory. At this level of investigation, the content of knowledge is thought by many to comprise four such categories:

1. Awareness of the existence of persons, things, places, events, processes, situations and similar phenomena. I can reasonably claim that awareness of my next-door neighbour, her car, her home, her career as a community nurse, the actual work that she has done and the circumstances in which she has done it, are all items that are numbered among the contents of my store of knowledge.

2. Awareness that 'something is the case'. It may be clearly the case that my neighbour is a highly competent and much respected nurse. These, too, are legitimate items in my store of knowledge, but they are items of a rather different kind, since the items in the first category were objective, factual items which could be observed and satisfactorily proved to exist by anybody other than a thorough-going sceptic, while items in this second category tend to be matters of subjective opinion, even if widely or universally held to be true.

3. Awareness of 'how something should be done'. Having spent hours talking to my neighbour over the garden fence, I may feel that I know a great deal about how to manage a confused elderly relative with decubitus ulcers, but the fact that I never had to do this or, having tried, have fallen far short of generally acceptable standards of care, suggests a fourth category of knowledge.

4. Acquisition of proficiency or even expertise, as defined above, together with something which we can describe more succinctly as the 'knack' of performing a practical task smoothly and without fault. This is a feature that cannot be described in detail in a textbook or lecture or even in audio-visual form because it requires hands-on experience over a long period of time to acquire this knack. We are now in the realm of psychomotor skills rather than of pure knowledge, even though once we have become proficient we do habitually say: 'I know how to manage the decubitus ulcers of confused elderly people'. This area of 'knowledge' is more appropriately considered under the heading of 'Skills'.

All four categories of knowledge add up to describe what Kenneth Boulding has named our 'image' of the world.[3] Without necessarily proving the reality of things, cases and methods, and without necessarily setting limits to what may be regarded as knowledge, the individual usually allows her image of the world to dominate and shape her behaviour as she reacts to whatever she perceives around her. The meaning of a message from outside may be regarded as the nature of the change which it produces in the recipient's image of her world. This is the whole point and purpose of any educational process: to ensure as far as possible, that the messages received from, or bounced off, the teacher however arranged or transmitted, are such as to procure the mutually-agreed or contracted changes in the student by slowly building up, and causing her to adopt, a particular image of that part of knowledge in which she is being educated, and react accordingly.

The teacher and the student have to bear in mind that there are considerable pitfalls in the communicating and absorption of knowledge and that transmission and reception are seldom completely efficient or comprehensive. Almost invariably, the teacher has to build into his communication some compensations for this loss: deliberate repetition or redundancy, consistent and logically-arranged sequences of material and other forms of eye- and ear-catching emphasis. The units or packages of knowledge and information which we create and pass on in this way are *concepts*. These are simple, unitary ideas about things and other phenomena which should approximate as closely as possible to the truth as far as it is known, and which are designed to serve a useful purpose. They are generalisations, arrived at by a process of abstracting or distilling the essential central element from a number of separate examples of a phenomenon. We have already identified and examined some concepts of mankind, society, health, ill-health and nursing care in our consideration of the philosophy and model of nursing.

As is usual in the pursuit of knowledge, we have built up these simple concepts into connected and related networks of *statements* which have extended the meaning of our concepts and helped to forward our overall purpose. They suggest, for example, that man has personality, dignity and worth simply because he or she exists and does not have to earn respect, love or the right to autonomy as an individual or the right to be cared for when autonomy breaks down.

Some eleven concepts have been built up here into a statement, resulting in a significant and, for us, true *proposition*. Supported by our own system of general beliefs, by our experience and by the form and persuasiveness of its expression in words and, perhaps, in actions, this proposition could now form the foundation for the study of a complete subject area of the health sciences in which we could move freely to create, arrange and organise knowledge, redirect it and extend it and predict the probable consequences of so doing, including the possibility of finding it to have been a false proposition all along. This could not be proved experimentally and must therefore be placed in the second category of knowledge: 'awareness that something is the case', rather than in the first category that can be proved by research and experiment.

With regard to *subjects*, we can no longer accept the former view of a subject as a unified and self-contained 'slice of the cake of knowledge'. This view asserted that a specialist in a subject could, by virtue of perseverance, learn the whole of his subject and be regarded as an authority, but at the same time, perhaps, remain woefully ignorant of other subjects. Today, it is realised that knowledge in a subject such as nursing is inextricably bound up with knowledge in other subjects, some directly related, some not so closely related, such as psychology, medicine, sociology, human and general biology, law and ethics, management and so on. The two views may be represented in diagrammatic form and it is instructive to bear in mind this picture of the field of knowledge as some professionals, including librarians, have to recognise and deal with it. The old idea of a subject may be best represented by Figure 9.1(a) whereas in present-day circumstances, a subject might be represented by Figure 9.1(b).

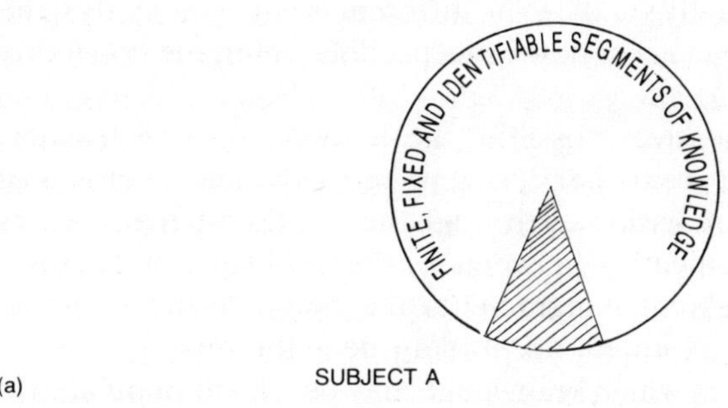

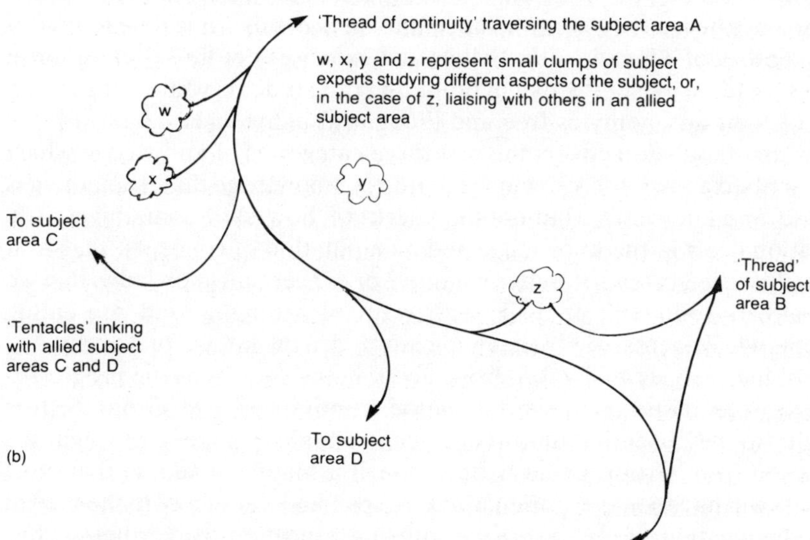

Figure 9.1 Two views of the concept of 'a subject'. (a) Old idea. (b) Present-day idea.

Concepts, being the building blocks by which knowledge is constantly created, arranged, rearranged, organised, redirected and extended, are capable of being manipulated in many different ways for these purposes, at many different levels of complexity. Each concept is a highly individual package of an idea, together with its related perceptions, associations, memories and emotions, which interprets some feature of the world in a quite unique manner. It may be shared or rejected or modified by other people and it is small wonder that, although we can produce a standard list of the ways in which it may be manipulated, the outcomes of manipulation will be as numerous and as varied as the manipulators. Many of the different outcomes will be almost equally valid – to be different is not necessarily to be wrong, although the introduction of new concepts does entail the possibility of introducing new errors.

It is important that, whenever possible, the learner, not the teacher, should do the manipulating at first hand, otherwise the beneficial effects of the learning will be diluted or dissipated through the less-than-perfect means of transmission and communication between teacher and student and also, as Burnard points out, the essential ingredients of experience and reflection may not be added to the mix unless the student does the mixing.[4]

The standard list of ways in which knowledge may be thus manipulated in the process of learning in order to effect changes in the learner has already been encountered in the first part of this book in which the whole process of curriculum design was reviewed in outline. It is reproduced as Table 9.1 for convenience because, as we concluded on that occasion, 'it is time to review the inventory of educational activities and exercises before selecting those which should be most effective in preparing our students while not robbing them of their autonomy as free and thoughtful individuals'.

This first tabulation covers the first three categories of knowledge which are described above: the knowledge of things, knowledge that 'something is the case' and knowledge (but not the knack) of 'how to do something'. The tabulation deals in the knowledge and manipulation of concepts, that is, it covers this three-category area of cognitive or conceptual knowledge that we have already outlined. It deals with ways of arranging and presenting concepts which increase in their complexity and in the intellectual extent and value of the changes which they bring about in the student as she progresses through work based upon the tabulation from Group 1 to Group 6. It is thought to be essential that the student should progress through the tabulation from Group 1 onwards, although it may be assumed that most students will have some experience of Groups 1 and 2 at school in the field of general education, if not in terms of nursing education. Nevertheless, this must be clearly ascertained and the re-alignment to nursing made smoothly and effectively by ensuring that the student performs and masters the prescribed educational exercises from the second column of the tabulation in the area of Groups 1 and 2. These are designed to create and encourage the development of curiosity about things and their names (1.1) and gradually turn it into the ability to identify current conventions and routines (1.4), trends in development (1.5), networks or classifications of related

Table 9.1

Knowledge	Column 1	Column 2
	The student should:	The student would show mastery of this when she:
1. Know about things:		Distinguishes things from each other
	1.1 Terminology	Defines things
	1.2 Facts	Recalls facts
	1.3 Means of dealing with things	Makes rules for dealing with things
	1.4 Conventions	States and describes conventions
	1.5 Trends	States and describes trends
	1.6 Categories of things	Recognises things as belonging to groups of things
	1.7 Criteria for categorising things	Classifies things into groups
	1.8 Methods and procedures	States and selects procedures
	1.9 Principles and generalisations	Discusses principles
	1.10 Theories	States, describes and compares theories
2. Comprehend knowledge		
	2.1 Translate ideas	Simplifies ideas in her own words
	2.2 Interpret ideas	Demonstrates and explains ideas
	2.3 Predict ideas	Infers and predicts on the basis of what is already known
3. Apply knowledge		Applies knowledge to a task
		Revises knowledge for a new situation
		Formulates proposals for development
4. Analyse knowledge		Distinguishes, compares and contrasts elements in a situation,
		Draws an organisational plan or flow-chart
5. Synthesise knowledge:		
	5.1 Produce an original text	Writes a useful summary of a topic derived from various sources
	5.2 Produce a plan for action	Writes instructions for carrying out a cooperative procedure
	5.3 State the relations in a situation as they are thought to exist	Carries out a minor piece of research and makes a report
6. Evaluate knowledge		Uses external criteria to judge a piece of knowledge as valid or not valid and selects or creates the criteria for judgement
		Criticises constructively and may go on to reconstruct and rearrange that piece of knowledge

concepts (1.7) and the procedures and methods (1.8) whereby the student can arrive at principles and theories (1.9) about the contents of her area of study.

All this preparation is believed to be necessary before the student can proceed to Group 2 and carry out further exercises to enable her to demonstrate comprehension of the concepts by translating (2.1) and interpreting the ideas involved (2.2) and even predicting (2.3) where they are likely to lead her investigations and learning.

With comprehension comes the ability to apply the newly-acquired knowledge of the concepts (3.0). Exercises from column 2 at this point show the way in which knowledge, once comprehended, can be invested in practical experience. Groups 4 and 5 specify ways of achieving much higher levels of intellectual appreciation of the concepts by breaking them down into their component parts (analysis 4.0), examining and plotting their organisation and working relationships and then reassembling, recreating or replacing the knowledge which they represent (5.0). In much the same way, a young engineer might be required, as part of his learning, to examine and then strip down a carburettor of a design which is new to him, reassemble it, build a replica of it or even design and build an improved version. In the manipulation of knowledge about things, of knowledge 'that something is the case' and of the theoretical knowledge of 'how to do something', the student is achieving the intellectual level of innovative research, on however small a scale. With the mastery of critical evaluation of her acquired knowledge and her own work in the Group 6 exercises, the student has now reached the ultimate intellectual level of self-critical research and the ability to assess critically and helpfully the work of others which may be submitted for her consideration.

From this point, as far as the knowledge and handling of concepts is concerned, there are no more techniques or procedures to be learned: the only remaining challenge lies in the increasing complexity and scale of the subject matter which is represented by the concepts to be managed. It is not, of course, necessary to go through this chain of exercises with every concept studied, but only to ensure that the course of study as a whole involves the students in these exercises, in this order, as it unfolds from beginning to end. If, by planning these exercises into your curriculum at appropriate points, according to the subject matter, and in sufficient quantity and variety, you have brought your students to the peak of achievement described above, you may regard your curriculum as successful. It is not possible to prescribe from outside a school or department exactly the right timing, mix and scale of these exercises because this is a matter for your own judgement and adjustment in the light of your philosophy, model and resources; an outsider can only show you the map and point out the road.

The nature and importance of attitudes

Attitudes may be regarded as the expression of personal values, that is, learned and fairly consistent reactions towards a person, object or situation.

Some examples of such values are caring, loving, being reliable, self-motivating, self-disciplined and innovative. Some values are best expressed in a negative way — refraining from condemning people, refusing to divulge confidences. They may be exhibited or carefully concealed by the owner and may vary in usefulness and effectiveness according to the situation — they may be a positive hindrance in certain circumstances. Conversely, they may be affected by particular situations, such as the learning/teaching process as defined by the formal and informal curricula that control it. A profession could seek to promote useful and worthy values and attitudes and discourage those that are useless or actually damaging to itself and its clients: one may query the feasibility and ethics of doing so.

In this way, values and attitudes may be clarified and, perhaps, modified, in order to achieve a clear statement of professional aims to which students can commit themselves for guidance in their daily work. Abstractions though they may be, values and the attitudes which give expression to them may be detected if the observer is perceptive and sensitive to the interpretation of body language and other signs and as long as the owner of the attitudes is not desperately anxious to conceal them. However, detection and interpretation are not easy. An observer, knowing something about another person, such as the nature of his work or his educational background, may all too readily abandon acute observation and realistic interpretation of what he sees of that person's attitudes for the short cut offered by the commonly-held stereotype of, say, the bank-manager, farmer or ex-soldier. Such 'implicit personality theories' are dangerous and those of us who have to spend much of our working life in assessing people, or 'weighing them up', need to have our prejudice scales calibrated from time to time.

This assessment is particularly important in nursing in view of the emphasis currently placed upon the centrality of the client and the nurse-client relationship in nursing care. Many vital decisions may depend upon this crucial assessment, although you might argue that if a nurse is to value a non-judgemental attitude vital decisions should not hinge upon such assessments and it is alarming to encounter Cook's conclusion that people are, for the most part, very inept at this.[5] Miller speaks of the difficulty of having only one criterion by which to judge attitudes – that of overt, observable, behaviour – if one is to discount voluntary self-reporting by individuals as being too much open to deception, even self-deception in many cases.[6]

It is especially dangerous when a nurse or other professional carer, makes a wrong assumption about the attitudes of a client upon inadequate evidence or fails to subject that evidence to a separate, confirming test. This is very likely to set up an uncharacteristic reaction in the client who may understandably feel annoyed or frustrated at being diagnosed as 'not deaf at all' by a nurse just because he made a rather brilliantly successful attempt at lip-reading the charge nurse's well-articulated words of welcome to the ward, and in spite of the prominent note on his records. That confrontation may well escalate and create unnecessary unhappiness and confusion for the duration of the client's stay or even for the duration of the nurse's career.

The more formal methods of detecting attitudes are equally hazardous in many respects. They are far from reliable, involving as they do the client's more or less willing cooperation as owner of the attitudes in question. Problems are raised initially by a number of people on both sides of the divide who object strongly that a person's attitudes and the underlying beliefs and values are a purely private concern. Although it may be grudgingly accepted that a teacher may be justified in manipulating a student's concepts or in persuading the student to manipulate her own concepts for her own benefit, the revelation, charting and manipulation of values, beliefs and attitudes for the benefit of others cannot be justified because, it is alleged, this is an unwarranted intrusion upon privacy. It is also objected that the investigation of attitudes has unfortunate effects upon those who are investigated, increasing their stress and reducing their self-confidence. It is even suspected that those doing the investigation are seldom at ease in their work.

In spite of these reservations, more formal methods of detecting and measuring attitudes may be brought into play and the fact that attitudes may change or be changed more rapidly and decisively than is thought possible by most people, makes it even more necessary to keep on monitoring such a potentially volatile situation by the most readily available and easily applied methods. Structured interviews, or more usually questionnaires on standard proforma, with built-in checks on the veracity of the respondent, may be imposed upon the person being investigated with, perhaps, only perfunctory gestures towards securing his consent, or, more deliberately, may be imposed upon his associates, relatives, teachers, or a selection of his peers. The individual may be required to respond spontaneously to some kind of stimulus as in the well-known Rorschach Ink-blot test, or to sessions on the lines of 'What's the first thought that comes into your mind when I say 'sleep'?'.

'Attitude scale inventories', of which there are several well-authenticated examples in print, comprise statements covering a wide range of general beliefs or attitudes regarding a particular subject, arranged in a random order and offering no clue as to what might be expected of the respondent by the investigator in the way of answers. The individual under investigation is then invited to indicate his reactions to the various statements in the test and an assessment of his attitudes is then derived from a point-by-point analysis of his answers in comparison with those of the large, randomly-selected 'jury' who validated the scale when it was first constructed.

The 'Repertory Grid Technique' is based upon the concept of the average person as being sufficiently intelligent to seek to understand and control the surroundings by rational experimental behaviour, and to predict trends and events, by preparing a series of personal constructs or hypothetical pictures of the present and future for his own guidance. It is the analysis of these constructs as they are proposed by the respondent for application to his relationships with friends and associates that is believed to give an insight into his own highly individual attitudes and to distinguish them from those of all other people, according to its designer, George Kelly.[7]

Even assuming that one has the necessary specialised education and training to do so, it is one thing to attempt to assess attitudes, however imperfect, approximate and error-strewn the attempt, but quite another to try to *change* them by means external to the 'victim' without his full cooperation. The history of the world from the most ancient to the most modern times is full of heart-rending accounts of atrocities committed for this end by investigators driven to extremes by the resistance of committed individuals.

Ribeaux and Poppleton offer a number of suggestions supported by research findings from the world of business administration.[8] They use variations on the basic structure of the communicator (attempting to change the attitude); the communication used; the situation in which the attempt takes place; and the 'target', the person whose attitude is to be changed. The presentation here is a simplification of their reports but is a basically useful abstract.

The communicator's prestige is an important factor: the greater his prestige the greater the effect of his persuasive powers; the greater his apparent honesty, the closer he approximates to the target in his background and life-style and the more likeable he makes himself, the more effective he is likely to be. The easier he finds it to subvert the target's peer-group and get them working for him, the more easily the target's resistance is undermined. However, if these forces do not achieve the desired effect fairly speedily – over a matter of a few weeks, perhaps – their influence fades and has to be constantly renewed.

The communication itself is crucial. It appears that where the communicator is not well regarded and the communication is at considerable variance with the target's earnestly-held convictions, increasing efforts to persuade meet increasing resistance. On the other hand, if the communicator is respected and the topic is not vital to the target's convictions, the communicator is likely to succeed however much his view might differ from that of the target.

In the case of the manner of the communication, intelligent targets are more likely to respond to discussion and to the deliberate omission of firm conclusions by an apparently open-minded investigator and to the presentation of an apparently new and untried message. Less intelligent targets are more likely to respond to a somewhat hectoring monologue, heavily reinforced conclusions and the reiteration of what they believe they know already but have been reluctant to admit.

The situation can be manipulated to the communicator's advantage. Pleasurable surroundings are persuasive; the arousal of fear, although not necessarily crude threats of physical or psychological violence, and the subsequent exploitation of either relief when threats are removed or of the aggression when threats continue unabated, can be very persuasive; distractions may secure the target's cooperation by deflecting his attention and concentration, as long as the communicator succeeds in getting his message through in the first place.

Finally, as regards the target himself, he seems to be more easily persuaded if he has a low opinion of himself and is of generally lower intelligence. Women in these categories have even less resistance than men, unless things have changed since this research was done in 1959![9] Targets appear to have different methods of countering persuasion, probably reflecting personality differences. One type is logical, aggressive and seeks to discredit both the communicator and his presentation by reasoned argument; the other type tends to be illogical, emotional and evasive and tries to pretend that nothing untoward is happening, but remains vulnerable to cunningly exploited insights.

Lastly, commitment and support are important factors for the target. If he is substantially and publicly committed to his attitude he is unlikely to change, especially if the evidence is that he took up his stance voluntarily and without external pressure. Support for him may take the form of either a mock attack on his beliefs, giving him then time to assemble counter-arguments, the so-called dry-run or inoculation approach, or it may be considered more helpful to supply him with ready-made arguments. Rather surprisingly, the former method of support is generally the more effective. It is not expected that you would ever stoop to, or even condone, such Machiavellian manoeuvres and this compassion for the target is perhaps yet another hall-mark of the professional worker. The 'Tabulation of Attitudes', which is reproduced as Table 9.2 for your convenience, is constructed in a similar manner to the 'Tabulation of Knowledge' in that the student is expected to master the initial and subsequent groups of exercises (column 2) and thereby master their associated attitudinal achievements, in the order in which they are set out. The basis for this sequence of learning is that it is unreasonable to expect a person to respond to a value (2.0) before she has become aware of it (1.1) and offered (1.2) and directed (1.3) her attention towards it and thereby received it. Similarly, it is difficult to imagine anyone committing themselves to a value (3.3) before they have received it (1), made an initial response (2) and come to accept (3.1) and indeed prefer (3.2) that value. In the final stages, it is hoped that the person will analyse the nature of the value (4.1), incorporate it into her way of life (4.2) and

eventually absorb it to the extent of unselfconsciously becoming characterised by it: a living manifestation or symbol of the value (5).

Table 9.2 Table of attitudes.

Attitudes	Column 1	Column 2
The student should:		The student would show mastery of this when she:
1. Receive (i.e. attend to):		Recognises something (e.g. a problem)
1.1 Become aware of		Takes heed (e.g. of a problem)
1.2 Become willing to pay attention		Shows sensitivity to something
1.3 Control attention		Selects an important element (e.g. a problem), observes it and is able to maintain attention
2. Respond:		
2.1 Acquiesce in making a response		Complies with a request to pay attention and participate
2.2 Become willing to respond		Volunteers to pay attention and to participate
2.3 Find satisfaction in responding		Enjoys the activity of responding; shares it with and recommends it to others
3. Value:		
3.1 Accept the value under consideration		Supports and adheres to, e.g. a belief
3.2 Prefer the value		Chooses this belief above others and prefers it to the state of not having a belief
3.3 Make commitment to the value		Defends it and refutes the opposite belief: works for its acceptance by others
4. Organise values:		
4.1 Conceptualise a value		Analyses ideas and creates a personal statement of the theory behind a belief
4.2 Organise a value system		Places the belief in the context of supporting beliefs and ideas to create a 'way of life'
5. Become characterised by a value or value system		Adopts a belief: changes to conform to it; adheres to it; applies it consistently; evaluates it and if satisfied, resists further change and assumes responsibility for the consequences

The curriculum designer who wishes to ensure, as far as possible, that the
students acquire new attitudes or reinforce acceptable existing attitudes that
will improve their lives and the lives of colleagues and clients, and who is
prepared to actually specify or negotiate what those attitudes should be, may
then build into the curriculum the necessary educational exercises (Step 7) in
the sequence indicated in column 2, associate them at a later stage with

related subject matter and ensure that they are reproduced, rehearsed and repeated as necessary in the lessons that are eventually planned (Step 8).

The nature of skills

It was tentatively suggested earlier in this book that the commonly-used expression 'nursing skills' as a means of describing all the nurse's contributions to her work, should be replaced for our present purpose, by another expression: nursing 'tasks'. It was desired to retain the word skills for the things that nurses can be seen to do for their patients in the course of their work as opposed to those elements of knowledge, attitudes and other attributes which they offer but which are not visible in action. Hence we have already prepared in Step 4 a list of nursing tasks and a parallel list of midwifery tasks, both of which encompass far more than manual or intellectual skills. Now the time has come to look more closely at skills in this narrower sense. It is important at the outset to distinguish two kinds of skills, even within the limits of the term as it has just been defined.

There is, firstly, the skill involved in such activities as counselling, interviewing, teaching patients, and documentation, in which there is a large component of 'knowing about', 'knowing that something is the case' and 'knowing how to do something'. There may well be a considerable contribution to success by the presence of appropriate attitudes, for example, in counselling, where empathy and objectivity may both be desirable. In so far as the overall product of these characteristics appears to be something of a hybrid with mixed parentage in the sectors of knowledge and attitudes, the situation is complex. It is made even more complex by the fact that it is undeniable that in counselling, for example, there is a clear need for skills that must be learned, practised in role-play or by some other means, and deployed in the real-life counselling situation in contact with a client. Since these skills are the most readily available and observable evidence that counselling is in progress, even though they may be barely distinguishable from the techniques of ordinary serious conversation, it seems appropriate to consider them in this section.

These skills will be referred to as 'intellectual craft skills' to distinguish them from purely manual skills or psychomotor skills. In the latter, training in dexterity and precision in the observable performance of physical tasks such as catheterisation or laying up a dressings trolley appears to obviate the necessity for knowledge of principles or adoption of particular attitudes, although these must indeed play an important part, especially if some kind of problem should arise involving, for example, the improvisation of equipment or the reassuring of an apprehensive client. Burnard refers to both categories as 'practical knowledge' though continuing to assert that there are skills 'not necessarily of a psychomotor kind'. He goes on:

A considerable amount of general nursing activity is generated out of the domain of practical knowledge. It is important to note, however, that a person may develop considerable practical knowledge without necessarily developing the appropriate propositional (that is, 'conceptual') knowledge. Thus, I may become skilled in giving an injection without necessarily knowing why I am giving it and without knowing the possible consequences of my actions. Again, it is probably better that practical knowledge is combined with a sound knowledge base from the propositional domain, but it does not necessarily have to be the case.

From this he draws the conclusion that nurse education up to this point has been dominated by propositional knowledge in the school-based blocks and by practical knowledge in the wards and in the community services. He attributes to this dichotomy the apparent gap in coordination which is said to exist between the schools and the service sectors.[4]

It appears to be the case that the two kinds of practical knowledge: the intellectual craft skills and the psychomotor skills, might be amenable to the same kind of analysis. Although nearly all the research in this area has been done in the investigation of psychomotor skills in industry or in the laboratory, it may be feasible to translate many of the ideas into the intellectual craft skill environment by interpreting such terms as 'performance', 'operator' and 'feedback' in a figurative, rather than a literal, sense without losing their essence. In this spirit, we can say of skills in general that until the period of the Second World War, they were regarded merely as the outward and physical manifestation of the response of a person or laboratory animal to a stimulus which might range from the promise of a larger pay packet to the anticipation of a trickle of birdseed or the desire for the warm glow of self-satisfaction. All of these, in their various contexts, would constitute a reward for adequate performance by the operator, and the feedback to the operator, once he had been rewarded, would be likely to set up a chain of stimulus–response reactions until the reward lost its attraction or the birdseed ran out.

This simplistic view was replaced after wartime experience of the skills needed to control very complex machinery, by a new emphasis on the importance of the feedback of the results obtained by the exercising of a particular skill to its human or mechanical or electronic operator as an influence which would not be regarded primarily as evidence that a reward was on the way but which would induce a self-regulating equilibrium in the system. Under this regime, the operator works more flexibly and responsibly; there is a future aim or overall purpose, rather than merely the promise of immediate reward, and there is a concern for economy and efficiency in pursuing it. Whatever the stimulus that triggers or maintains the performance of a skill, the nature of skill itself has been defined by Ribeaux and Poppleton as:

the performance of any task which, for its successful and rapid completion, requires an improved organisation of responses making use of only those aspects of the stimulus which are essential to satisfactory performance.[8]

Problems have arisen over the speed, precision and dexterity with which highly skilled workers operate in the field of psychomotor skills. They are said to work, on occasion, many times faster than they could if they had to wait for the operation of a human stimulus-response or feedback mechanism, since visual and information-processing and muscular reaction times are far too slow to keep pace with the actual output of work. It has been suggested that stimuli, feedback and responses are anticipated in a routine task such as typing, packaged together, as for example in units of words, phrases or whole sentences in copy-typing, and triggered by a single impulse — a matter of habit inculcated by training rather than of the application of painstaking skills.

The *acquisition* of skills follows a similar pattern. There are suggestions that acquisition is a three-stage process: a cognitive or knowledge-based first stage in which the operator is brought by discussion and negotiation to understand what is needed and how to achieve it; a stage in which the stimuli in the task are identified and responses to them are planned during guided practice; and a final stage, analogous to the achievement of expertise, in which the skilled actions are so successfully modified and rehearsed in the course of experience by the increasingly effective interpretation and use of feedback, that little conscious control is needed and the delays due to even relatively speedy reaction times are virtually eliminated, subject to the intervention of such human feelings as stress or fatigue.

A debate has centred round the question as to whether it is better to learn a skilled procedure as a whole or in a series of cumulative steps. To help to determine this, skills have been analysed in two dimensions: one describing the number of different parts or stages in the performance and their individual complexity and the other describing the complexity of the relationships or organisational structure in which the parts are set and in which they operate. It has been suggested that a task which is in many parts, only loosely associated with each other, could well be learned in parts or stages, while a task comprising closely-knit sequences of activity should be learned as a whole for maximum efficiency. A different division of the elements of the task into levels with a succession of goals and sub-goals to be achieved facilitates the adoption of the learning-as-a-whole approach in the case of repetitious skills such as grading fruit, while a strategy can be evolved on the lines of an algorithm or flow-chart in the case of such tasks as fault-finding on a piece of machinery.

The last of the three parts of the 'Table of Learning', that dealing with the psychomotor skills of manual operations, especially those using equipment,

Table 9.3 Table of practical skills.

Practical skills[12,13]	Column 1	Column 2
The student should:		The student would show mastery of this when she:
1. Exhibit reflex movement		Reacts spontaneously and instinctively to a stimulus
2. Exercise guided manipulation or imitative manipulation		Follows, simulates or copies a task or the steps of a procedure
3. Exercise independent manipulation by trial and error rehearsal		Operates equipment, lifts or turns a patient etc. under supervision only
4. Increase in precision generally Increase in precision of:		Practises to perfection
	4.1 Coordination	Synchronises movements
	4.2 Sequencing	Performs activities in the right order
	4.3 Consistency	Responds regularly and correctly and maintains consistency of output
5. Attain proficiency in:		
	5.1 Skill	Performs accurately
	5.2 Dexterity	Performs with speed, precision and accuracy
	5.3 Acquisition of 'natural' performance	Performs with smoothness, evenness and accuracy
	5.4 Automaticity	Performs spontaneously and accurately and with control
6. Adapt by:		
	6.1 Improvisation	Overcomes adverse factors by adapting procedures without prior planning
	6.2 Modification of environment	Rearranges setting, or –
	6.3 Modification of skill	Reorganises skill strategy to overcome adverse factors
7. Experiment and innovate		Tests, develops and implements improved skills, settings, etc. without immediate pressure to adapt
		Considers whether or not the skilled operation is still valid in the light of new knowledge or changed circumstances

is reproduced as Table 9.3. It does not specifically include reference to the intellectual craft skills of interpersonal relations or the special skills involved in such non-manual operations as documentation or checking temperatures where no particular psychomotor skills need be involved other than the almost universal abilities to attend, write and interpret digits. Nevertheless, you should consider whether or not these *non*-psychomotor intellectual craft skills can be analysed and learned by the use of this tabulation if their specification and exercises are translated out of the language of the psychomotor domain into more appropriate terms without destroying their meaning or relationships.

As before, the tabulation leads the student towards higher-level attainment. At the lowest level is the skill of responding spontaneously to a stimulus such as a tap or a wave (1), but the student is soon expected to move through a phase of guided or imitative hands-on manipulation of whatever device is involved (2) and through trial and error attempts (3) with gradually increasing precision and smoothness of operation (4 and 5) to controlled spontaneity (5.4) and eventually to the familiarity which enables her to cope with problems by modifying or improvising devices and procedures (6) and going on to design and test completely new ones, or even to declare the skill redundant if the circumstances warrant it (7). The student is expected to walk before she tries to run in this area too.

In Step 7 we shall proceed from the vantage point of our increased acquaintance with the nature and promotion of knowledge, attitudes and skills to see how an appropriate mix of these ingredients can be made up into a prescription for an educational objective. This package will ensure, as far as possible, that the student who works her way through to the achievement of that educational objective will, in the process, become the right kind of person, with the necessary or desirable attributes, to perform the task to the maximum benefit of everybody concerned.

References

1. Benner, Patricia, From novice to expert, *American Journal of Nursing*, March 1982, Vol. 82, No. 3, pp. 403–407. Also reported in *American Journal of Nursing Guide*, 1987, p. 31.
2. University of London, Kings College, Department of Nursing Studies, *Report of the Nursing Process Evaluation Working Group: Chairman: Phyllis Friend; Editor: Jack Hayward* London, 1986, Nursing Education Research Unit, Report No. 5.
3. Boulding, Kenneth, *The image*, Ann Arbor, University of Michigan Press, 1956.
4. Burnard, Philip, Towards an epistemological basis for experiential learning in nurse education, *Journal of Advanced Nursing*, March 1987, Vol. 12, No. 2, pp. 189–193.
5. Cook, M., *Perceiving others: the psychology of interpersonal perception*, London, Methuen, 1979.
6. Miller, Audrey E., Nurses' attitudes towards their patients, *Nursing Times*, 8 November 1979, Vol. 75, No. 45, pp. 1929–1933.
7. Kelly, George A., *Psychology of personal constructs*, New York, Norton, 1955, 2 volumes.
8. Ribeaux, Peter, Poppleton, Stephen E., *Psychology and work: an introduction*, London, Macmillan, 1978.

9. Janis, I.L., Field, P.B., Sex differences and personality factors related to persuasibility, in Hovland, C.I., Janis, I.L., (editors), *Personality and persuasibility*, New Haven, Connecticut, Yale University Press, 1959.
10. Bloom, B.S., *et al.*, *Taxonomy of educational objectives: classification of educational goals: Handbook I Cognitive domain*, New York, McKay, 1956.
11. Krathwohl, D.R., Bloom, B.S., Masia, B., *Taxonomy of educational objectives: classification of educational goals: Handbook II Affective domain*, New York, McKay, 1964.
12. Simpson, E., *Classification of educational objectives: psychomotor domain*, Urbana, University of Illinois, 1966.
13. Harrow, A.J., *Taxonomy of the psychomotor domain*, New York, McKay, 1972.

Further reading

Kemp, D.A., *The nature of knowledge: an introduction for librarians*, London, Bingley, 1976. (Librarians are the professionals who have the task of understanding, organising and presenting knowledge).
Fenton, Mary V., Development of the scale of humanistic nursing behaviors, *Nursing Research*, March/April 1987, Vol. 36, No. 2, pp. 82–87. (Does not purport to measure attitudes but to quantify the care-oriented functions in a unit that may express attitudes.)
Fielding, Pauline, *Attitudes revisited*, London, Royal College of Nursing, 1986, RCN research series.
Warren, Neil, Jahoda, Marie, editors, *Attitudes: selected readings*, 2nd edn, Harmondsworth, Penguin, 1973.
Legge, David (editor), *Skills: selected readings*, Harmondsworth, Penguin, 1970.
Department of Education and Science, Further Education Curriculum Review and Development Unit, *Basic skills*, London, DES, 1982.

Chapter 10

Step 7   Educational objectives: specifying appropriate knowledge, attitudes and skills and the accompanying educational exercises for each nursing task

Reminder

The treatment of this step in the 'Brief Outline' chapter ran to several pages and you might be forgiven for thinking that there can be little more to say on the subject. In order to make a start, however, it may be desirable to summarise the purpose of that section, which was to demonstrate how to set up an *educational objective* as part of a series based upon and co-extensive with the list of nursing tasks which was constructed in Step 4. One should remember that in this context, 'tasks' is a word to be interpreted broadly rather than in a narrow, literal, sense.

Each educational objective should be a statement so framed as to cover one or more of the tasks – or in some cases, perhaps, only a discrete part of a task — and to express exactly what it is that the student has to achieve and be assessed upon, to indicate that she has, in fact, attained the objective and mastered the task as one more step in her professional education. Each educational objective carries with it a unique package comprising a statement of the elements of knowledge, attitudes and skills which you consider to be necessary for its attainment (from the 'Tabulation of Learning', column 1) and a parallel statement of the type of educational activity required for the learning of each of those elements (from column 2).

An example of such a package, dealing with the preparation of a dressings trolley, was included in Step 7 of the 'Brief Outlines' chapter at the beginning of this book and is reproduced in this Step for convenient reference. It is a small, but fully worked out and rather complex, perhaps even over-complex, example, but it should help you to follow the rest of this Step with more understanding.

Task: To prepare a basic dressing trolley and prepare the patient for dressing a
wound.

Educational objective for the achievement of this learning:
While under the supervision of a tutor or clinical teacher in the practice ward,
the student will state clearly the reasons for the procedure; will select and lay
out on the top and bottom trays of the trolley as appropriate the full range of
necessary basic items; will prepare the 'patient' by explaining the procedure,
screening, positioning and reassuring the 'patient' and exposing the dressing
site. Changes sought: to plan and execute procedures with care. This task will
be assessed by the supervisor who will award one mark for each item or part of
the procedure correctly dealt with up to a maximum of 25 marks. Marks will be
deducted at the rate of one per minute for time spent on the procedure in
excess of 10 minutes. A score of 20 marks or more will be regarded as evidence
of success at this stage of the course.

In order to obtain some idea as to how this might be translated into actual
academic exercises in the 'class-room', you might find it useful to note that
the principal relevant *activities* from Step 6 might perhaps, be as follows:

Knowledge: of things (1.2), facts (1.2), conventions (1.4), methods and procedures (1.8), application of knowlege (3)
The student can identify the trolley and its contents, recall and apply the
knowledge of the conventional layout and the procedures of laying out the
trolley and preparing the 'patient'.

Attitudes: controlling attention (1.3), making commitment to a value (3.3)
The student can concentrate on the task in hand and feel a determination to
ensure the comfort and well-being of the 'patient' committed to her care.

Skills: Attainment of proficiency and dexterity (5.2), improvisation (6.1)
The student should exhibit, at this stage of the course, a reasonable degree of
dexterity in handling the equipment and the 'patient' and should be able to
improvise a solution to problems created by an unsatisfactory environment,
for example, poor light or an overcrowded ward.

The exercises listed in the right-hand column of the tables in Step 6 against
these activities, or at least an appropriate selection of them, would then be
woven into the lessons planned in Step 8 to teach this task, with the virtual
assurance that if the curriculum be well-designed the successful student
would be both competent in preparing the trolley and 'patient' and would
also be the best kind of person to accompany a real patient through a
possibly distressing experience.

At the end of this Step you, as the curriculum designer, should have a
schedule of educational objectives in this pattern, together with their related
educational activities, for the whole curriculum. They will not yet be in any

particular order or formation, not yet loaded with subject content in the final form, nor with recommendations for methods of learning, teaching or assessing, but they will be ready for the addition of these features in Step 8 and will offer an essential framework for their placing.

It should be understood that from this point onwards a textbook such as this, written by an outsider, cannot and should not attempt to specify what *you* need for *your* students in *your* school or department, even if you have accepted the philosophy and model of nursing offered in previous steps. You are now on your own and, although the book can offer this framework, a method and some examples, you must now fill in the details in each of the remaining steps, if only as an exercise for your own instruction.

Aims, goals and educational objectives

You will, no doubt, have heard of aims and goals in connection with curriculum design and development and this is a matter that should be clarified now. To anticipate slightly the points to be made later about objectives, one might say that in their formulation you should always make precise and quite detailed specifications as to what the student should achieve in order to demonstrate mastery of each objective. Expressions such as 'Acquire a concern for...' or 'Develop self-critical faculties in respect of...' are not suitable for the specification of educational objectives but are only very broad aims or goals for the whole educational process and not appropriate for specifying how to achieve an individual task within that process.

This introduces the distinction, which must be drawn initially and carefully maintained throughout the design stages, between the broad aims and goals of education for nursing and the much narrower, much more specific and detailed educational objectives which, together with their individual learning packages, we are now concerned to establish for each task of nursing which we have enumerated in Step 4. You will find that many textbooks on curriculum design, especially those produced for use in the general schools for the education of children, refer to the derivation of aims and, perhaps, several layers of goals as a series of successive stages of expansion towards the eventual specification of educational objectives. For our present purpose this would appear to be an unnecessarily long and complex approach to the process.

To take first the matter of educational 'aims', these usually amount to three or four statements which, between them, may be regarded as a very broad and perhaps somewhat sketchy overview of the purposes of the proposed course of education as seen by the curriculum designers and teachers. It would appear to be very difficult to produce any meaningful guidance for teachers and students in such a complex and skilled area of study as education for nursing within these brief confines. Any such statement would have to be couched in terms so bland and generalised as to lack any substantial message upon which action in education of any degree of originality could be based.

It could be regarded only as a set of recommendations about the general drift or character of a course, rather than as a basis for action, revolving around such self-evident issues as the production of well-motivated, caring nurses, their acquisition and mastery of techniques, promotion of social skills and the provision of incentives to pursue continuing education as a lifelong activity. Aims are, perhaps, of somewhat greater value in such settings as post-basic and other short courses where the main issues may be submerged within the general aims of nursing as a whole and therefore less self-evident than in basic education.

However, since we have observed that the education for nursing as a whole is inextricably linked with the *vocation* of nursing to such an extent that under many regimes the two proceed in parallel, each seeking simultaneously to serve the purposes of the other, there is every reason why we should regard the philosophy and model of nursing itself, which we have specifically constructed for our purpose of curriculum building, as a completely adequate set of aims for our guidance. There can be no valid reason, at the level of aims, for desiring any further guidance or defining any more closely our responsibilities to students. It is here, in the philosophy and model of nursing itself, that our purposes have, not only their roots, but their whole being, and where they will exert the maximum encouragement and reassurance and inspiration on new learners. These are the permanent pillars of nursing and they stand above the ebb and flow of changes in techniques and other relatively minor matters which will affect the validity only of the more detailed and specific educational objectives.

You will also come across extensive discussion in some quarters of educational 'goals'. Indeed, the term is sometimes used in place of both 'aims' and 'objectives' and this is quite unpardonable, especially within the same book! It may be helpful in some circumstances to include a consideration of goals as an intermediate step in the process of narrowing down the definitions of purposes from broad aims to specific objectives and some writers go to the extent of recommending the gradual refinement of purposes through two or even three stages of broad ultimate goals, slightly narrower mediate goals and rather narrower and more numerous proximate goals, each step representing an expansion of detail and definition over its predecessors. These might be regarded as broadly corresponding with the three levels of Butler's 'Taxonomy of competences'[1] which is organised upon the lines of our adaptation of the 'Tabulation of Learning' in that the attainment of each level in the hierarchy assumes that the student has mastered the preceding 'lower' levels. The hierarchy comprises:

1. Generic (basic) competences: simple skills which are fundamental to all everyday human activities, such as the use of rules and procedures to carry out tasks.
2. Definitive (global) competences: skills for lifelong development as required by students in further and higher education, such as skills of learning, self-awareness and most social skills.
3. Enabling (educative) competences: the knowledge and skills through which students can attain and demonstrate the definitive competences (2 above) and the ability to carry out professional and similar tasks within the remit of the definitive competences, and the attitudes which they imply.

Butler maintains that the totality of these competences, as chosen for inclusion in the curriculum design, will reflect and define the aims and goals of the institution which frames them.

You may find a use for this categorisation of competences but to use them to underpin a three-fold, or even single, set of goals in a field with which you are already completely familiar as a practitioner, seems to be a needless extravagance and a waste of time and other precious resources which are in short supply. In any case, the use of goals in this way is a convention which, one suspects, is more honoured in the breach than in the observance. You would be well advised to keep it simple and go straight from the philosophy and model of nursing which you favour to the listing of tasks and the delineation of corresponding detailed educational objectives as specifications for the changes to be wrought in the students through the learning of those tasks. However, you have now encountered the terms *aims* and *goals* and you will have some ideas about their significance and value to you as a curriculum designer.

The role of the tabulation of learning in formulating educational objectives

Before we look more closely at the nature and uses of educational objectives, it might be appropriate to make a bridge between the previous Step, Step 6, in which we looked at knowledge, attitudes and skills in their 'pure' state, and this Step 7, by reviewing first the ways in which the 'Tabulation of Learning' in those three areas could be of great assistance, and may, indeed, be indispensable, to the curriculum designer in the practical business of making educational objectives.

Some teachers, when asked to describe the outcome which they hope their students will achieve at the end of a course or even a single lesson, use very vague terminology which is in everyday conversational use but which does not convey any clearly defined or measurable description of achievement by which their own efforts and those of their students can be interpreted and assessed. Many anticipate that their students will 'come to understand the subject' or even 'really understand' it; that they will 'appreciate its significance in modern society' or 'grasp the essentials' of it or perhaps only 'become acquainted' with it. These expressions of intent are so imprecise as to be almost meaningless and might equally be achieved by any kind of learning, from a five-minute briefing or a half-hour video recording right up to a four-year research-based doctoral programme. They are, as we have seen above, broad aims at best. It is difficult to imagine what these teachers mean and how anyone else could possibly cooperate with or complement their efforts.

The 'Tabulation of Learning' assists by enabling curriculum designers to help teachers to specify quite precisely the desired and expected end result of the learning that is to take place. For example, it offers any one of more than a dozen different ways of 'knowing' or 'understanding' a fact or collection of facts: all of them individually identifiable and measurable. Furthermore, it lists and explains to the curriculum designer, teacher and student, a wide field of different ways of learning these outcomes. This helps to introduce variety into the course and it thereby minimises boredom and considerably increases the efficacy of the process. For any one piece of learning there may well be half-a-dozen almost equally valid pathways to the summit. All the student's efforts may be directed into one route; alternatively, several different routes may be tried in rapid succession to achieve an all-round view, or this may be spread throughout the duration of the course in the manner of a spiral curriculum, each reinforcing and perhaps extending the learning achieved under its predecessors. This varies the aspect and the approach, keeping up the momentum of the learner's progress and offering new challenges from time to time. It enables students with different talents to make an effective effort in those particular academic styles in which they may feel particularly confident and capable, while still offering them exercises in other styles of learning.

From the teacher's point of view, teaching methods can be varied by taking advantage of the 'Tabulation's' suggestions in column 2 for a variety of educational exercises, all of which contribute to a single achievement or a small package of related achievements in teaching and learning. The curriculum designer must become accustomed to exploiting this variety of approaches and methods, ringing the changes and seeking out the most appropriate means or selection of means for achieving a given objective, in the light of the talents and tastes of a particular group of students or even of an individual student or teacher. Above all, perhaps, there arises the question as to how anyone can have any idea about when the learning is completed and how effective it has been, apart from having a hunch that all is, or is not, well. How is it possible to assess the achievement by a student of 'real understanding' or 'appreciation of significance' except in the broadest and least satisfactory terms? This could be done only by submitting students to some kind of survey, interview, examination or other means of assessment which would have to be equally vaguely worded, which might be at complete variance with their legitimate expectations and for which they might be unable to prepare themselves since they would have no precise knowledge of the purposes for which they had been taught. How deep is 'understanding'? How broad is 'appreciation'? How readily can these dimensions be measured for acceptably precise and helpful assessments to be made? The 'Tabulation of Learning' offers a way out of all these difficulties.

Educational objectives in the three categories of learning

One hesitates to break an established convention in the order in which topics are presented but it may be easier to dispose first of the educational objectives in the category of *Skill-learning* since these tend to be the most clear-cut and precise. Educational objectives are held by some authorities to be valid *only* when they are designed to produce, and to be judged by, the clearly observable behaviour which accompanies and identifies the perform-ance of a well-rehearsed physical skill with a quantifiable, and therefore easily assessed output of a given standard. Such a skill might be the making of a row of empty beds, where there is no complication involving the much less clear-cut factors of interpersonal relations with the occupants of those beds. Programmed texts in book or machine-based form, are, in general, most succinct and successful when they teach, or rather 'instruct', the user in some such clear-cut, skill-based technique which is amenable to the multiple-choice method of learning, although successful programmes have been produced in such abstruse areas as the study of the nature of knowledge itself without compromising their essentially logical reasoning structure. The fact that it is not easy to think of a nursing task that involves *only* the application of manual skills suggests that the characterisation of nursing as an 'intellectual craft profession' is not far short of the mark.

However, much of the earlier insistence upon strictly and literally observable and measurable behaviour as the only permissible outcome of the application of educational objectives has now been dropped, even in the case of skills-learning, in deference to the common-sense view that many perfectly proper and useful objectives cannot be made manifest in overt measurable behaviour on the part of the student even in the most favourable circumstances. While not accepting the vagueness of an objective such as 'really understanding how to make empty beds', there are yet ways of expressing an objective which are adequately demanding to the student and rather more amenable to the determination of success or failure, even if not to the more precise measurement of outcome, in common-sense terms quite suited to the needs of a profession such as nursing. It is possible, for example, to use some such device as a two, three or five-point scale for grading the learner.

Nevertheless, an appropriate degree of precision is relatively easy to define and specify in formulating educational objectives for the psycho-motor skills of nursing, such as they are, and there should be little or no difficulty in following and emulating the example of setting a dressings trolley which has been offered in this book. In the sphere of cognitive educational objectives for the attainment of *knowledge*: 'knowledge about something', 'knowledge that something is the case' and 'knowledge of how to do something', we move into an area of somewhat greater complexity in that a fact, unaccompanied by a network of supporting facts, definitions and explanations to put it into context, is no more than a bare word and should be learned as a concept with its supporting context and evidence.

In the first place, different kinds of knowledge bring with them their own differing criteria as to what is authentic proof of achievement and what degree of accuracy of assessment is appropriate for a given purpose. Generally speaking, modern thought and teaching are accused of requiring far more accuracy than is likely to be of use in many circumstances: a reasonable degree of rounding or approximation in some kinds of assess-ment may be acceptable rather than the pursuit of the tenth place of decimals: some relaxation of the more irksome aspects of grammar, such as the pursuit and exposure of neat, concise, perfectly clear and manageable, but undeniably split, infinitives, is probably to be welcomed where mis-understandings are likely to seldom, if ever, arise. Much knowledge is the product of arbitrary decisions, conventions and reluctance to re-think, extending back over many decades. The rules of punctuation and of the representation of music in print or manuscript, are examples of phenomena which one might hesitate to perpetuate in their present forms in a curricu-lum, given the opportunity to start afresh from the beginning, were it not for the pressures of tradition.

Even in the case of scientific knowledge, stemming from the confirmation of hypotheses based upon observations, experiments and tests and cumu-lated over many lifetimes, we find that much knowledge was relevant only to a particular theory, now discredited or developed beyond its original form until virtually unrecognisable. It is therefore the responsibility of the curri-culum designer to examine closely the kinds of knowledge and the relevance of the current 'received wisdom' in many aspects of nursing and to break fresh ground if the departure from the norm can be justified in the light of current research findings and clients' needs. This is one important way of ensuring that properly validated and evaluated research, that has been shown to prove what it set out to prove and is actually useful in practice, is implemented without delay.

Whatever the decisions that are reached in these matters, it is important that the knowledge to be offered to the students should be selected for its relevance to their needs and the needs of clients, rather than being harvested uncritically in an attempt to be comprehensive. A new curriculum is an opportunity to eliminate uncertainties about what might or might not be needed, in the relatively short run of basic education at least, so that precious time and effort are not squandered in the process of education. The degree of detail and the way in which it is organised within the curriculum is crucial for the same reasons. A major function of the educational objective and its formulation is the review and reorganisation of knowledge in this way as a recurring activity.

Having assembled a body of knowledge to be absorbed by the students, in the terms suggested by groups 1 and 2 of the 'Tabulation of Knowledge', the curriculum designer should ensure that it is not allowed to lie fallow until required for regurgitation in some kind of memory game masquerading as an examination. The recipients must be persuaded to use their newly-acquired knowledge in practical or simulated applications as in group 3 of the Tabulation. In particular, they must be given opportunities to manipulate their ideas by breaking them down into their constituent concepts and reinterpreting, re-arranging and re-assembling them into new combinations and contexts in the search for new approaches to contemporary problems, as in groups 4 and 5 of the Tabulation. The further presentation, discussion and self-critical viewing of these approaches on however small a scale, is probably the highest achievement which you can offer to your students in this intellectual or cognitive part of the Tabulation. It appears to be a major deficiency in many candidates for the Diploma in Nursing, a major cause of their often-expressed dissatisfaction with the course and a major cause of the distressing sense of inadequacy which some feel. A post-basic course of that kind is no place to catch up with the rudiments of intellectual analysis, synthesis, research and development.

As regards the question of educational objectives in the affective area of *Attitudes* in nurse education, everybody working in this area is at a disadvantage. Very little has been done to examine systematically these phenomena or make firm recommendations about the formulation and evaluation of the range of objectives for teaching and learning about attitudes and feelings in higher vocational education. Similarly, little effort appears to have been made in most curricula to follow up the initial enthusiasm for changing and developing attitudes by actually building the necessary features into the formulation of the relevant educational objectives and thence into the relevant teaching, learning and assessment procedures. This has already been made evident in the case of curricula for post-basic studies in some institutions, which tend to include the appropriate sentiments in their introductory paragraphs dealing with the philosophy and model of the proposed course, but thereafter to launch even more enthusiastically into the more familiar and comfortable practicalities of the subject with scant regard for earlier pious professions of concern.

Much of this neglect probably stems from the difficulty of detecting and especially of grading such changes in the student, even on a simple two, three or five-point grading scale. Another difficulty arises from the students' apparent ability to exploit the vagaries of trial-and-error learning by first identifying and then relentlessly mimicking those elements of behaviour which are found to meet with the teacher's approval. It is very difficult to distinguish this from a genuine change of attitude and most assessors tend to abandon the attempt after one or two initial skirmishes. There is also the problem, already noted, of the genuine reluctance of many individuals to reveal their attitudes and of the genuine anger that many feel when required to do so in pursuit of a qualification to practise. Such a qualification might thereby be interpreted as a reward for submitting to a degree of indoctrination rather than as the outward and visible sign of an inward achievement gained under an educational regime that should be a model of the democratic exercise of choice and voluntary cooperation with the institution and its objectives.

As has been suggested before, attitudes can change or be changed quite suddenly and dramatically, contrary to popular belief – at least, the outward signs of conversion often seem to appear rather unexpectedly. This might suggest that, instead of being the slowly developing fruit of the long-term acquisition, interpretation, breaking down and restructuring of knowledge into new patterns, attitude change may, in some cases, be the product of the pursuit of specially formulated educational objectives, based upon the analysis of feelings, emotions and intuitive reactions, which may be just as effective in their own sphere as the educational objectives which are designed for the attainment of knowledge itself. As in the case of factual knowledge, attitudes have to be placed into an elaborate network of concepts, definitions and explanations before they can come alive for students.

Much may be done in this matter by the examples of 'wholesome' attitudes and 'appropriate' overt behaviour on the part of teachers, librarians and other members of the staff of a school or department, and of course, staff in the service sectors, too. This is particularly influential when joint appointments or link-tutor schemes bring education staff into contact with clients in the wards, clinics and community where students are also present. Carefully framed educational objectives may serve to direct the students' thoughts and attention to such matters, even if it proves difficult to use these objectives to 'teach' and 'assess' in these affective studies. The rather alarming possibility is raised that the teacher might not be able to demonstrate the students' achievement of objectives at all. Many of these problems revolve around the quality described by Taba as 'intangibility':

> The term 'intangible' conveys a suggestion that these objectives are inherently incapable of being fully understood, hence also incapable of serving as a focus for teaching, learning and evaluation. An adequate behavioural analysis of these objectives would dispel this notion.[2]

Suffice it to say that no such behavioural analysis appears to be adequate for this function at the moment. Any progress we make here will be strictly our own.

Perhaps this is a suitable point at which to reiterate a remark already made: this three-fold division of educational objectives into the categories of knowledge, attitudes and skills is largely a matter of academic convenience. It reflects an important but rather over-emphasised feature of curriculum design. In practice, it will be found that tasks, objectives and prescriptions for learning and teaching tend to blur these crisp outlines in so far as they may cater for more than one of the categories at a time; as a curriculum designer, it is part of your function to identify and exploit these occasions and the opportunities which they present for economy and reinforcement in construction.

The formulation of educational objectives: some background factors

Objectives have several vital functions to perform in curriculum design and development which we have already discussed in passing but which might be conveniently summarised here. Firstly, from the teachers' point of view:

1. Objectives prescribe how, in favourable circumstances, the students should be changed by their educational experiences which are being designed for that specific purpose. In the present case, the student should be changed in the direction of professional competence based upon acquired cognitive and manual skills, together with a substantial affective element, since it has been determined already that professionalism resides largely in standards and attitudes.
2. They are essential to the stages of planning the desirable learning experiences, subject content, learning and teaching methods, means of student assessment and the organisation and evaluation of courses, since they provide a framework upon which to hang and shape these activities with a minimum of duplication and ambiguity. They constitute an

economical and, above all, systematic, approach to curriculum design.

From the point of view of the students, the specification of each objective implies and requires five major elements:

1. The desirable changes in the students' behaviour.
2. The circumstances and manner in which these changes are to be exhibited and the clues by which they may be identified.
3. The means by which they may be assessed and the degree of competence which shall be accounted 'success'.
4. An element of intellectual challenge such that the students' expectations are fulfilled. Without this many, usually the best ones, feel cheated.
5. An element of the spirit and reality of 'creativity' which offers much in the way of motivation and which may well attract and hold the less intellectually gifted students as well as their more gifted peers.

It is important to gauge their reactions to the use of objectives in setting the direction of thrust, speed of advance, intellectual activities and levels, the content and day-by-day organisation of their studies. In the first place, many of them will not have encountered this approach to the definition of courses before, or will not have encountered its overt use nor been consulted about its design and implementation. Once the method has been explained to them and once they have been acquainted with the detailed description and sequence of the objectives, as should always be the case, it becomes the responsibility of everyone concerned to hold to the course as publicised.

It appears from the findings of an admittedly limited amount of research in this area, that students benefit from having advanced notice of what they should be attempting to learn, and that the intrinsic value of the objectives becomes all the clearer as each one is tackled in turn and as the consequences of failure and the rewards of success are made apparent. Cowan reports that first-year engineering degree students were dealt with in this manner and that ninety-three per cent understood the listed objectives of the course and could relate them day-by-day to the course content; approximately fifty per cent had used the list of objectives at least 'a fair amount' during and after classes and for revision purposes. Half of these had found that the efficacy of their study methods were changed for the better, also by 'a fair amount' and in the case of the other half, study had improved by 'a considerable amount'.[3]

There is also the advantage that in publicising educational objectives throughout the institution, supervisory nursing staff out in the wards, clinics and community are much more aware as to what to expect from students who are committed to their care at a given point in the course and can complement the efforts of the school or department much more effectively and smoothly.

It is still not possible for an outsider to specify with certainty the best formula for producing objectives to achieve any particular skill or competence in a particular institution. It is a matter for local formulation in the light of local needs and resources and for a period of trial and error and adjustment within that institution. It is possible for the outsider only to narrow the range of choice and to make recommendations as to priorities for use by teachers with unique skills, teaching students with unique needs. Eraut says:

> It is also important to emphasise that we know very little about teaching and learning; and the implication of this is that any course we design will be far from the optimum in its effectiveness. Nor will any further consultation with experts or searching of the recent literature be likely to result in any significant improvements. If due attention has been paid to what little is known about teaching and learning, trial and error becomes the remaining method of improvement.[4]

Similarly, it will not always be possible to predict what will be the outcomes of the educational process; the hidden curriculum is a very real hazard to curriculum designers. Nor will it always be possible to predict or even estimate to what extent they will fail to coincide with the expressed objectives of any institution. It may be that by suppressing all except those originally intended, much of real value may be lost. This is not an immediate concern here but it does bring up the need for constant review of the curriculum and its objectives after implementation and the possibility of having to select from among a superfluity of potential objectives unless a very generously open-ended regime is deliberately chosen. Wynne Harlen has stressed this point:

> Frequently a situation leads to learning which had not been anticipated, the outcomes more numerous and more complicated than could be encompassed by any reasonable set of objectives. When certain outcomes have been predetermined, it is felt that others, more numerous and possibly more valuable, may be strangled at birth.[5]

The formulation of educational objectives: specific factors

The construction of a range of educational objectives to cover the whole course and based immediately upon the agreed list of nursing 'tasks' appears to be a formidable undertaking. There is, indeed, no short-cut, no easy way to achieve what is needed for this next step of the curriculum design process. It is simply a case of sitting down, either as a complete design team or as a number of sub-groups or individuals with delegated sections of the list, and, for each task on the list, making a deliberate choice of the change sought in the students at that point, the objective which, when achieved, could bring about that change, the learning required to achieve the objective (from the 'Tabulation of Learning' (column 1), and the educational exercise or exercises that should enable the student to achieve the learning and attain the objective (from the 'Tabulation of Learning', column 2), and demonstrate the desired change.

There is little guidance that can be offered by anybody outside the group but you might like to consider how the following factors can be utilised. The *criteria* for the selection and formulation of educational objectives may be summarised as follows:

1. Credibility: Objectives must be such as to gain the students' interest and cooperation and must be within the capabilities of the average student while having the potential to stretch the best students.
2. Relevance: They must be of immediate and obvious value as contributions, not only to the course, but also to the clinical nursing service activities which lie beyond the course but still within the sights of the students. In scope, they should be relevant to situations which arise most frequently and occupy the most attention in educational and clinical practice and should preferably have transfer value to other related fields of health care and to the steady accumulation of general learning.
3. Accessibility: Broadly this refers to the institution's calculation of the cost-effectiveness of teaching to a particular objective in the manner recommended, in terms of time, staff, materials, library back-up and other resources.
4. Compatibility: Objectives must be formulated in the light of possible conflict with personal and institutional standards and those of society at large.
5. Utility: It is also necessary to consider the immediate uses and the degree of permanence of the skills and competences which are specified.
6. Impact: Curriculum designers must attempt to assess and exploit the likely effect of their objectives upon the students' motivation to learn and upon the whole range of attitudes which they possess at the commencement of the course and those which they are expected to acquire during the course.
7. Clarity: Objectives should be quite unambiguous in meaning and expression.

These criteria should be weighted and ranked in every case where conflict between them or within the curriculum design team suggests that a balance must be struck and a decision made.

In the next place, the philosophy and model of nursing formulated at the beginning of the process, must still be allowed over-riding influence on the spirit and substance of all that is produced, even down to the frequent use of their key-words and expressions. These should be constant reminders that you have already laid down unassailable boundaries and immutable guidelines by which you remain bound as long as you all agree upon the desired qualities of the nurses whom you are planning to educate, the qualities which are enshrined in these public statements. Further, you may be guided in your thinking by the data about the students which your school or department will have on file. You should be concerned to know their previous educational experiences and achievements, their general background, their needs and interests, the nature and problems of their contemporary life outside the institution, and the likely conditions, tasks, problems and prospects which they may encounter within the institution.

Next, educational objectives will tend to be shaped in accordance with the nature of the subject matter of the every-day practices of nursing which the list of tasks helps to define, much as a skeleton defines the outline of the body but requires the addition of much detail before it can be made to work. The nature of the subject matter will suggest networks of related concepts and sub-objectives. It may also suggest the making of links with other subject areas and related topics such as psychology, sociology and some basic sciences, because of their contribution to the wider background and professional interests of mainline nursing. The subject matter, although not the primary concern in shaping the student or her objectives, will nevertheless be influential in suggesting the kinds of learning that can be deployed to her advantage, as was noted in the preceding Step 6. At that point, we were examining the role of the 'Tabulation of Learning' which offers an overview of the kinds of learning, but not of course the subjects, which are both available and appropriate.

In this regard, the curriculum design team should also take into account some idea, however broad, of the kind of education envisaged for the students. It is, perhaps, unnecessary, although intensely interesting, to dig deeply among the many views on the psychological underpinnings of vocational education and this book is not intended as a primer of educational psychology. Suffice it to say that there are many intermediate points on the long spectrum between, at the one extreme, 'operant conditioning' which, quite respectably and legitimately for many purposes, uses rewards to convert the trial and error learning of people and pigeons into a form of habitual behaviour or indoctrination, and, at the other extreme, the method of 'pure' or more often, subtly guided, 'discovery learning' in which the student builds up a picture of a probable 'general case' or condition in an area of study from a series of individually discovered instances and then proceeds, again by trial and error, to her own generalisation about the situation, rather than that intended for her by the instructor.

Put like this, it is rather alarming to consider to what extent there is any significant difference between these two extremes, other than the degree of guidance involved, if the end-product is intended to be the assimilation of a defined package of learning. The former method is the speedier, more economical, more thorough, more cost-effective in resources and possibly more damaging to the student and is not usually recommended for learning anything except the most imperative and rigidly defined procedures. The latter is the more relaxed, more time-consuming, more expensive in money and other resources, but the more truly 'educational' and challenging method which, at the same time, respects the integrity and self-development of the whole person and therefore appears to reflect the ethos of nursing and of education for nursing in a way which is conspicuously absent from operant conditioning.

Finally, you could be guided to a large extent by your own experience in nursing, your own learning and teaching experiences and your professional reading. It has already been indicated in the discussion of the nursing philosophy and model that, in spite of the opportunity, and, indeed the obligation, to think things out afresh from the beginning, you may quite understandably arrive at conclusions that differ very little from those with which you started out. The closer this match, the more justified you may be in using your own experience as a guide in this new and more rigorous approach to educational processes. As part of this process of applying your own experience as a nurse to the formulation of educational objectives, you might consider it appropriate to take account of some variables relating to the intrinsic nature of the organisation of nursing and the tasks involved, as you have seen them and experienced them. Quite apart from the largely self-evident title and functions of the staff nurse, the actual tasks and the conditions under which they are performed may differ in different parts of the service sector and the educational objectives designed to educate nurses for those differing functions may need to reflect some of the special requirements. The curriculum is, after all, a *local* curriculum.

The variations which education might wish to reflect might include, for example, several degrees of autonomy in the selection of problems and in freedom to innovate; several degrees of the extent of the new nurse's influence within the organisation; several degrees of difference in the sources and consequences of the assessments made of her successes and failures; and a range of requisite or desirable personal attributes upon which she might be judged. You might regard some or all of these factors as being irrelevant to your local curriculum but a brief tabulation is given in Tables 10.1 and 10.2 in case you wish to take them into account.

Table 10.1 Tabulation of variables relating to the tasks of
nursing, adapted from J.L. Schofield.[6]

1. Degree to which the nurse identifies and selects problems for
   investigation on a scale of: (a) no autonomy to (e) full autonomy
2. Degree of freedom to innovate
   on a scale of: (a) no freedom to (e) full freedom
3. Nature of preparation for problem-solving and innovation:
   (a) requiring no formal specialised knowledge
   (b) dependent upon knowledge acquired 'on the job'
   (c) dependent upon a broad general education
   (d) dependent upon basic nurse education
   (e) dependent upon later post-basic education and training
4. Extent of the nurse's influence in her special role:
   (a) limited to her own service point
   (b) limited to her department
   (c) limited to her institution as a whole
   (d) extending to the Health Authority
   (e) extending to the general public in the community
5. Identity of those affected by her actions in her special role:
   (a) clients
   (b) manual and clerical staff
   (c) fellow professionals
   (d) executives of the institution
   (e) executives of the Health Authority
   (f) the general public in the community
6. Nature of the assessment of success or failure:
   (a) no assessment except self-criticism
   (b) informal assessment by clients
   (c) informal assessment by peer-group opinion
   (d) informal assessment by superiors
   (e) formal assessment by superiors
7. Consequences of 'failure':
   (a) personal threat to conscience and self-image
   (b) threat to relations with peer-group colleagues
   (c) threat to smooth running of the administration of the
        institution
   (d) threat to smooth running of services to clients
   (e) threat to the reputation of the institution

Educational objectives for learning the procedure for aseptic dressing technique

Firstly, the Procedure Instruction is reproduced in Table 10.3, followed in
Table 10.4 by the recommended educational objectives that might be
produced for the design of the relevant part of the General Nurse basic
education curriculum. These have been drawn up in the light of the criteria

Table 10.2 Tabulation of personal attributes related to the tasks
of nursing, adapted from Shropshire County Library
practice.[7]

1. Possession of sound motivation.
2. Possession of sense of responsibility.
3. Ability to lead with authority.
4. Ability to maintain good relations with all grades of staff.
5. Ability to maintain good relations with staff teams as groups.
6. Ability to maintain good relations with clients.
7. Ability to make sound professional analyses, judgements and decisions.
8. Ability to make good general analyses, judgements and decisions.
9. Possession of sound general professional knowledge.
10. Possession of sound knowledge of the institution and its procedures.
11. Ability to express ideas coherently.
12. Ability to give instructions coherently.
13. Ability to achieve satisfactory speed, volume and quality of output.
14. Capacity for original thought and innovation.
15. Capacity for involvement with continuing education.
16. Capacity for involvement with outside activities and community matters.

and recommendations discussed above and listed below, as they might be
expected to apply in a medium-sized school of nursing attached to a district
general hospital.

Check-list of criteria and recommendations

You should consider and specify for each educational objective:

1. Relevant elements of your philosophy and model of nursing.
2. The overall aim and goal.
3. The selection of a specific 'task' or 'tasks'.
4. Change(s) sought in the students.
5. Elements of knowledge, attitudes and skills required to bring about these changes ('Tabulation of Learning', column 1).
6. Educational exercises required to help students to attain those elements of knowledge, attitudes and skills ('Tabulation of Learning', column 2).
7. Criteria by which performance can be detected (if not overt).
8. Conditions under which performance is to be carried out.
9. Method of assessing standard of attainment.
10. Minimum standard for 'success'.

11. Contribution to the overall pattern of the course.
12. Link to the next educational objective.

You should look for means of ensuring:

1. Intellectual challenge.
2. Opportunities for creativvity if appropriate.
3. Effective, up-to-date and economical learning and teaching.
4. Credibility.
5. Relevance.
6. Accessibility.
7. Compatibility.
8. Utility.
9. Clarity.
10. Appropriate educational experiences for a given student or group (from the 'Tabulation of Variables and Personal Attributes').
11. Input from your own experience, if relevant.
12. Clear evidence of achievement by the students.

Table 10.3 Aseptic dressing technique: procedure instruction

Definition
Those factors which lead to general recovery and will produce a micro-environment associated with the wound that will allow healing to proceed at the maximum possible rate relative to the age and physiological condition of the patient.

Hazards
1. Dressings which are cut for use during the procedure can cause particles to be released to contaminate a wound.
2. Removal of dressings before a surgical round allows superimposed infection.
3. Dressings which have stuck to the wound may be freed by soaking with Normal Saline before being gently removed. Gauze is particularly adherent and careless removal can cause tissue damage and delay healing.
4. Wounds without discharge do not require cleaning. Dried blood along a suture-line acts as a protective barrier and should not be removed.
5. Antibiotic impregnated dressings may cause an unpleasant allergic response. It is advised that obtaining a prescription ensures medical instructions are clear whilst providing opportunity for discussion. Wound variation may require specific diagnosis and subsequent management regarding antiseptics/antibiotics.

Table 10.3 (contd)

Pre-procedure explanation and preparation
Before the explanation is given to the patient consider:
1. Your attitude and approach to the patient. You will need to be supportive, sympathetic, kind and sometimes firm. Remember to maintain the individual's dignity and privacy at all times throughout the procedure.
2. Is analgesia needed? Is it prescribed? Has it been given?
3. Timing: Is the patient generally comfortable? Has enough time been allowed for any analgesics that may have been given to become effective, as this will help tolerance of possible discomfort? Inhalation analgesia may be an alternative.
4. Explain the procedure to the patient in terms that he will understand, especially what will be seen, felt, heard or smelt. Remember this is a new experience for most patients. This rehearsal will help the patient to cope. Give the patient a chance to ask questions/express feelings so goal differences are resolved. Anxiety can reduce healing, increase pain awareness, prevent patient's cooperation, and even lead to depression.
5. Bear in mind the cosmopolitan population and language problems that you may encounter and use the official list of hospital interpreters if one is available.
6. Obtain verbal consent from the patient before the procedure.
7. Assist the patient to where the dressing is to be carried out if applicable.
8. Allow airborne organisms to settle: Close adjacent windows/remove potentially contaminated material (e.g. locker-bag, close and remove). Draw curtains (if safe to do so), ideally allowing ten minute interval.
9. Place the patient in a comfortable position, taking into account his/her general condition and site of the wound so that it is accessible for redressing.
10. Leave a blanket to hand to cover the patient in case it is required later.
11. Remember to utilise gravity if possible to ensure the dressing stays in position before being taped.

Preparation of equipment
1. Remove used apron, don a fresh one.
   Long nails, rings and untidy hair are a potential source of infection (see Authority Code of Behaviour).
2. Using paper towels and general purpose detergent, wash and dry trolley thoroughly if not done earlier. This trolley should never be used for any other purposes.
3. Before each dressing wash and dry hands (See 'hand washing technique') and spray trolley with Dispray No 2. Dry with a paper towel or wait two minutes until it is dry.

Table 10.3 (contd)

---

4. Equipment: Take only likely requirements to avoid wastage,
   placing same on the bottom shelf of the clean dressing trolley;
   check autoclave marks have changed on packs;
   reject torn or damp ones or those with old water-marks; check
   expiry dates (packs and lotions).
   Sterile dressing pack consists of:
   >   wool balls
   >   gauze swabs
   >   forceps
   >   dressing towel
   >   gallipot
   >   pulp tray for used instruments
   >   inner wrapper for sterile field

Sterile supplementary packs may be required, including
instruments (refer to patient care plan).
Fluids for cleaning-irrigation (e.g. Normal Saline) always check
expiry date.
Steret to clean lotion sachet.
Hypo-allergenic tape or a bandage.

If necessary
Sterile disposable polythene gloves for removing grossly soiled
dressing.
Plaster-removing agent and sterile gallipot.
Large strong paper bag.
If desired, sterile latex gloves, e.g. Triflex (cheaper than
Surgeon's) for a technique using gloved hands.

Procedure

1. Take trolley to patient, disturbing screens minimally.
2. Open outer cover of sterile dressing pack, carefully tearing along
   sealed edge; or peel open, sliding contents on to top shelf.
3. Clip disposal bag to the trolley rail below the top shelf (so
   contaminated material will be below the sterile field).
4. Open inner wrap ensuring inner surface remains sterile (handle
   corners only). Use forceps to arrange equipment and place pulp
   tray on bottom shelf aseptically. Place forceps so that the part
   handled is OFF the sterile field and away from the corners. NO
   potentially contaminated material must be returned to the sterile
   field.
5. Open sterile supplementary packs. (Opening out the packet's
   side-folds with the thumbs may assist minimal air disturbance
   during tipping out on to the centre of the field).
6. Cleanse lotion sachet with Steret and pour aseptically.
7. Without undue exposure of the patient turn the clothes back with
   minimal movement. Prevent cooling and maintain the patient's
   dignity.
8. Without handling the dressing, prepare it for later removal by
   loosening tape gently. Pressing the skin away from it, along its
   length, helps, or using plaster solvent.

Table 10.3 (contd)

---

9. Wash and dry hands.
10. Use forceps or sterile polythene gloves to remove the dressing into waste-bag; discard forceps into tray.
11. Carefully position the dressing-towel without flapping it around, thus reducing airborne contamination.
12. (a) Inspect the wound. If clean, do not swab (soggy tissues support bacterial growth).
    (b) Use one pair of forceps for swabbing only and another pair for contact with pack only. Prevent contact between them.
    (c) Similarly, use a dry or lightly moistened swab if wound is oozing. Do not wring out. (This prevents contamination from the swabbing forceps).
    (d) If it is necessary, swab cleaner parts of wound first.
    (e) Use each swab once only (minimising further contamination).
    (f) Clean from inside to outside of wound, e.g. down centre then each side.
    (e) Dry carefully, similarly, if lotion used.
13. Discard forceps used for cleaning into a tray.
14. Apply dressing with remaining two pairs of forceps: discard similarly.
15. Secure dressing with enough tape to prevent contamination/ leakage when the patient moves. Replace tape on bottom shelf, to avoid contaminating it. Apply bandage if necessary.
16. Make patient comfortable.
17. Place: opened unused dressings on top shelf unless the wound is contaminated; the folded up sterile field and the gallipot (if empty) into waste bag; (place a full gallipot into the instrument tray to avoid a leaking bag).
18. Close bag and re-attach to rail. (Placing it on the trolley potentially contaminates it.)
19. Draw curtains back.
20. Dispose of potentially contaminated waste-bag, instruments and sharps appropriately.
21. Wash hands.
22. Put away uncontaminated tape.
23.

IF WOUND CONTAMINATED	IF WOUND NOT CONTAMINATED
Discard all unused dressings (packed or loose).	Put sterile unused dressings away.
Wash trolley with Stericol 1% and dry.	Spray trolley with Dispray No 2.

24. Report/record condition of wound. Report missing items.

Ongoing care/education
1. Check whether the patient is clear as to what surgery has been performed (if applicable) and the reason. (It may well be advisable to involve a qualified nurse and/or doctor at this point.)
2. Warn the patient not to touch his wound or peep under the dressing, giving the reason.

Table 10.3 (contd)

---

3. Explain specific arrangements for wound care, including washing/ not washing the area.
4. Remind him to support an abdominal wound when coughing/ sneezing/straining at stool, whether it is sutured or not. (Application of steri-strips is an additional precaution.)
5. Before being specific, discussion needs to take place with the surgeon responsible for the case with regard to activities of living, e.g. bending and lifting.
6. Explain exactly what sort of activities should be carried out, and allow opportunity for questions, e.g. explain light housework, and clarify what activities you include.
7. Define which activities should be avoided and why. Relate this to the patient's usual commitments (including employment).

Table 10.4 Recommended educational objectives.

Overall aim
Section 11 of the 'List of Nursing Tasks' (Step 4): 'Practical implementation of nursing care: techniques'.

Subsidiary goal
Sub-section 5 of Section 11 of the 'List of Nursing Tasks' (Step 4): 'Deal with problems in...infection...preparation for and carrying out of procedures...'

Educational objectives: Set 17: Aseptic dressing technique

Task 1: The Preamble
The student will:
(a) State briefly in writing the special circumstances in which dressings of any kind must be carried out on behalf of a patient who is otherwise, in the terms of the Nursing Philosophy and Model, an autonomous and respected individual, normally both capable of self-care and also the subject of self-care promotion activities by the nurse.
(b) State briefly in writing the roles in which the nurse operates in the course of this task, as technician, communicator, carer, educator, deliverer of prescribed medical care.
(c) State briefly in writing the particular problem to which her problem-solving approach is to be applied in the case of aseptic dressing technique and her knowledge of any recent research findings which are relevant to the task and which should be recommended for inclusion in the procedure.
Changes sought in the student: orientation towards the planning of a 'set-piece' practical task involving a considerable degree of responsibility for a patient.

Tabulation of learning

Column 1:		Column 2: particularly:
Knowledge	1.1 – 1.10	■ Makes rules for dealing with things
		■ States and describes conventions
		■ States and selects procedures
		■ Discusses principles
	2.1 – 2.2	■ Explains ideas

Table 10.4 (contd)

| Attitudes | 1.1 – 1.2 | ■ Recognises and heeds a problem
■ Volunteers to pay attention and participate |
| | 3.3 | ■ Defends the value (i.e. the value of self-care but the supremacy of aseptic integrity) |

Conditions: 30 minutes library-based investigation; 10 minutes classroom-based discussion; 15 minutes for written presentation in note form.

Assessment method: one mark for listing and one mark for adequately explaining each relevant item.

Standard: minimum of (x) marks.

Contribution to the course: introduction to the concepts of aseptic technique: revision of main elements of philosophy and model of nursing: revision of dressings in general.

Link to next educational objective: presentation of criteria and circumstances of preparation for and application of aseptic technique.

Task 2: Preparation of the working area, patient, equipment and dresser(s)
The student will:
(a) Prepare a diagrammatic presentation of the hazards and counter-measures regarding the exclusion of sources and carriers of cross-infection from treatment room and ward.
(b) Demonstrate in role play the preparation of the 'patient' by explaining the procedure, counselling and transferring a helpless 'patient' to the treatment room.
(c) Demonstrate the preparation and loading of the dressing trolley in accordance with the procedure instruction.
(d) Demonstrate the cleansing and protection of her own person and clothing.

Changes sought in the student: awareness of the importance of well-planned and carefully executed preparation for any major task, especially one involving patients directly.

Tabulation of learning:

Column 1:		Column 2: particularly:
Knowledge	1.4 – 1.8	■ Defines things; states and describes conventions; classifies things into groups; states and selects procedures
Attitudes	3.1	■ Supports and adheres to the value of asepsis
Skills	2	■ Follows, simulates or copies a task or the steps of a procedure, then
	3	■ Manipulates under supervision
	4	■ Performs activities in the right order

Conditions: investigates and demonstrates with a practice trolley and equipment in the practice ward with a live 'patient'; approximately 10 minutes for each element (a) – (d).

Assessment method: grade on a scale of 0 – 5 for performing procedure accurately and in the right order, first under supervision and subsequently without the tutor's intervention.

Standard: minimum of Grade 5.

Contribution to the course: preparatory procedure for aseptic dressings; learning the need for the use of procedures in tasks generally and for the use of appropriate equipment; learning the importance of thorough preparation; revision and reinforcement of the concepts and attitudes concerned with caring for vulnerable apprehensive patients.

Table 10.4 (contd)

Links to next educational objective: rehearsal of preparations for the activity of aseptic
   dressing.

Task 3: Execution of aseptic dressing in accordance with the procedure instruction
The student will:
(a) Carry out a briefing of her 'assistant dresser', describing the complete procedure with
   the aid of her own flow-chart.
(b) Demonstrate the appropriate placing of the equipment in relation to the 'patient' and
   open up and arrange on the trolley all the items to be used.
(c) Demonstrate the reassuring and positioning of the 'patient' and the removal of an old
   dressing with maximum regard to the integrity of the aseptic conditions and the
   comfort of the 'patient'.
(d) Demonstrate the inspection and cleansing of the 'wound' in accordance with the
   simulated condition which she discovers or the fictitious condition devised and
   described by the tutor.
(e) Demonstrate the application of a clean dressing.
 (f) Demonstrate care for the patient's comfort and show competence in ensuring a safe
   return to the ward; advise on self-care.
(g) Demonstrate the checking and disposal of the trolley and all equipment and supplies.
(h) Complete a fictitious set of records relating to the event and make all necessary
   reports to the tutor who acts as ward-sister/charge nurse.
Changes sought in the student: orientation towards low-level leadership skills; careful and
   methodical deployment of her knowledge of 'how to do something', attitudes of caring
   and skills of manipulating different categories of equipment and supplies; thorough-
   ness and legibility in compiling and presenting records and reports; coherence and
   clarity in verbal presentations.
Tabulation of learning

Column 1:		Column 2: particularly:
Knowledge	1.1 – 1.10	■ States and selects procedures
	2.1 – 2.2	■ Demonstrates and explains ideas
	3	■ Applies knowledge to a task
	4	■ Draws an organisational plan or flowchart
	5.1 – 5.2	■ Writes a useful summary
		■ Produces instructions for carrying out a cooperative procedure

(Aim in subsequent 'spirals' of the curriculum to include 6 – criticises constructively and
may possibly reconstruct this piece of knowledge.)

Attitudes	1.1 – 1.3	■ Shows sensitivity to something or somebody
	2.3	■ Enjoys responding, shares it and re-commends it
	3.3	■ Defends the value of asepsis and works for its promotion
	4.1	■ Analyses ideas and creates a perso-nal statement of the theory behind a belief in asepsis

Table 10.4 (contd)

Skills	2	■ Follows, simulates or copies a task
	3	■ Manipulates under supervision
	4.1	■ Synchronises movements
	4.2	■ Performs activities in the right order
	5.1	■ Performs accurately

(Aim in subsequent 'spirals' of the curriculum to include 6.1 – student overcomes adverse factors by adapting these procedures by improvisation. 6.2 – 6.3 – she modifies environment and skill as necessary.)

Conditions: (a) – (g) should be demonstrated with the practice trolley and equipment in the practice ward, working in pairs with a live 'patient'. Time available should be as long as necessary to learn to the standard required, bearing in mind local organisational constraints. Another opportunity must be sought for 'assistant dressers' to carry out a briefing in some other context and for 'principals' to record and report if, as is recommended, pairs change roles after completion of stage (d).

(h) may be carried out in the classroom: approximately 10 minutes allocated.

Assessment method: grade each pair on a scale of 0 – 5 for performing procedures accurately and in the right order, including a consideration of the adequacy of briefing and recording and reporting.

Standard: minimum of Grade 5.

Contribution to the course: this marks the completion of students' first complex practical procedure in intimate contact with a 'patient'; revision and reinforcement of the need for the use of procedures and of adequate preparation; revision and reinforcement of the concepts and attitudes of caring; learning the need for careful briefing of assistants and careful and accurate recording and reporting.

In the case of this last sub-objective for task 3, there may or may not be a link with the next educational objective, since it comes at the end of a discrete section of the curriculum. (See also Tabulation on pages 143 and 158.)

You will, of course, devise your own layout and short-hand symbols for all these different elements of an educational objective since most of them will recur time and time again throughout your growing curriculum. You may not feel the need for this degree of detail in the specification of objectives in any case but beware of omitting stages and elements which you might later need as foundations for some other objective or at some other level of the curriculum 'spiral'.

We have spent a long time on the discussion of educational objectives because the completed list of objectives in the pattern indicated forms the crux of the whole procedure of curriculum design. It represents the culmination in an 'operational plan' of all the thinking which you have put into the Nursing Philosophy, the Nursing Model, the Nursing Process, the List of Nursing Tasks, the Philosophy of Education for Nursing, the

Tabulation of Learning and into the consideration of Knowledge, Attitudes and Skills. At last, you can see your curriculum coming to life. From this point, having crystallised this operational plan in outline, you have only to clothe it in subject content and recommendations for learning, teaching and assessment methods, and then tailor the resulting curriculum to fit the organisational framework of your own school or department. It will then be ready for validating to ensure, as far as you can foresee, that it will deliver the product that you have specified, and after that you will feel free to implement the final curriculum.

References

1. *Butler, F. Coit. The concept of competence: an operational definition, Educational Technology*, January 1978, pp. 7–18.
2. Taba, H., *Curriculum development*, New York, Harcourt Brace World, 1962.
3. Cowan, John, Student reaction to the use of detailed objectives, *Aspects of Educational Technology*, Vol. 6, Proceedings of the Bath Conference, 1972, pp. 272–276.
4. Eraut, Michael, Course development: an approach to the improvement of teaching in higher education, *Journal of Educational Technology*, October 1970, Vol. 7, No. 3, pp. 195–206.
5. Harlen, Wynne, Formulating objectives: problems and approaches, *British Journal of Educational Technology*, October 1972, Vol. 3, No. 3, pp. 223–236.
6. Schofield, J.L., Job evaluation, job analysis, job satisfaction and resistance to change, *Library Association Record*, October 1975, Vol. 77, No. 10, pp. 241–243.
7. Shropshire County Library, Professional staff assessment form, *Library Association Record*, January 1975, Vol. 77, No. 1, p. 4.

Further reading

Beard, Ruth M., Healey, F.G., Holloway, P.J., *Objectives in higher education*, Society for Research into Higher Education, Working Party on Teaching Methods, London, SRHE, 1968.
Beard, Ruth M., Hartley, James, *Teaching and learning in higher education*, 4th edn, London, Harper & Row, 1984, Ch. 2, pp. 24–43.
Hinchliff, Susan M. (editor), *Teaching clinical nursing*, 2nd edn, Edinburgh, Churchill Livingstone, 1986, Ch. 4, pp. 81–96.
Marson, Sheila N., *Guide to developing self-instructional materials*, 3rd edn, Sheffield, English National Board Learning Resources Unit, 1983, pp. 41–61.

Chapter 11

Step 8 Allocating subject content and methods of learning, teaching and assessing to lesson units

Reminder

The ultimate purpose of this curriculum design process is the production of a special kind of person for the special function of giving nursing care to people who cannot cope with their own physical or emotional health problems for the time being.

The approach to this end has involved deciding what nursing *is*, what are its methods and tasks, what kind of educational activities are available and how they can be put to work to produce the right kind of person with the right resources of knowledge, attitudes and skills.

Subject matter has not been at the forefront of our thinking so far, but has rather tended to accrue around the task-based educational objectives in more-or-less appropriate packages simply because the concept of each task necessarily implies some kind of nursing content or activity to give it identity and substance.

It is now time to carry out the following operations:

1. Ascertain whether or not all necessary subject content has been included in your Tabulation of Educational Objectives and edit the tabulation by adding whatever might be needed and eliminating unwanted duplication, remembering that some 'redundancy' can be of considerable value.
2. Organise the educational objective packages into an appropriate sequence of modules, lessons and other groupings such as foundation, core and spiral curriculum units, to fit the organisational and timetabling constraints of the school or department.
3. Recommend learning, teaching and assessment methods for each

objective-based lesson, or, alternatively, make it clear, if necessary, where lie the limits of the individual teacher's autonomy in such matters.

It is not the function of this book to discuss and make firm recommendations about content, organisation or methods. It does not set out to supplant any of the admirable texts that already exist to cover these areas of education and a brief selection of these is offered in the further reading list at the end of this Step. It is to these that you should turn for information on these matters which, while very important in themselves are, in a sense, peripheral to the central concerns of curriculum design and development.

The designation of subject content

The designation of the subject content of any educational programme is normally the process which arouses most interest, particularly since it comes at the end of a long gruelling slog through the drafting of some two or three hundred educational objectives and gives the design team a glimpse of their haven at the end of the road. It is commonly regarded, of course, as being in itself the totality of curriculum design instead of, as we are now aware, a relatively late stage in a process whose foundations take so long to establish.

The subject content of nursing is necessarily volatile in the light of a general re-thinking of the roles and functions of nurses; the implementation of new systems of leadership and management; the introduction of new technology; and the need for a wider remit of nursing studies, especially in the social and psychological sciences, which may be of particular importance in the context of the removal of some nursing education to universities and polytechnics. Above all, perhaps, we are aware of the emergence, through the agency of nursing philosophies, models, and the machinery of the Nursing Process, of a distinct professional entity with its own sphere of operations and its own distinct responsibilities complementary to, but not subordinate to, those of medicine and the special therapies and sciences.

It is taken for granted that the curriculum will be presented as a unified whole which will accommodate all general nurses, many of whom will, no doubt, depart to specialised fields in midwifery, paediatrics, theatre work, dual general/mental health qualification, occupational health or teaching, after appropriate post-basic education. This appearance of 'wholeness' or general comprehensiveness may give the impression that there is no end to the list of subjects for inclusion in the subject content of nursing, no limit to the knowledge and skills which a nurse might be expected to command. A number of factors tend to modify this view and restore some degree of perspective and scale.

In the first place, the basic list of nursing tasks drawn up under the control of the philosophy and model sets limits to the expansion of the curriculum by presenting a finite list of related basic themes and key concepts which form the network known as 'nursing'. The process of control is strengthened by the disciplined manner in which educational objectives are derived from the same basic list of tasks, with primary consideration being given, not to a spread of subject matter to be learned but to a relatively small number of advances on the narrower front of changes sought in the students. Subject content is metered into the curriculum to fuel these changes rather than to present merely a list or syllabus of specified content to be taught.

There is a further limiting factor in so far as this type of curriculum is integrated, that is, it forms a self-contained and self-sufficient entity with no loose ends and no unattached codicils. The tendency in some educational regimes, particularly in North America, is to respond to a new or newly-expanded topic by adding another module or optional extra to the course. This 'add-on' proliferation does, in fact, get out of hand very readily, whereas a more fully integrated course such as that recommended here would absorb the additional knowledge in its appropriate context without undue extension of the curriculum. This could be done, for example, by teaching a set of principles which could be applied to different contexts, including the new one, rather than by teaching a possibly endless series of relatively small units of factual knowledge or techniques, one for each nursing context to be considered by the course designers.

In all these matters, the control by the philosophy, model and list of tasks must be pre-eminent since that is the main reason for their application to curriculum design, but it is only fair to admit that some elements of this thinking and planning stem from the traditions, predilections and intuitions of the individual curriculum designers in a particular institution, working within a particular organisational framework and set of resources. However, a subject or discipline such as nursing gains its unity from its own internal logical development of the knowledge basis which it requires, the skills which it teaches and fosters and the attitudes which it evokes and which affect the ways in which it is perceived by its practitioners, teachers and students.

It is sometimes claimed that the mere presentation of the subject content will cause a properly-motivated learner to be mystically transformed by the discipline which the content is said to exert upon the mind, irrespective of the nature of the process of learning. The whole message of this book is that the nature of the process of learning is itself the formative influence, and the subject content, though important in vocational studies, acts in the process of education substantially as a vehicle for the presentation and mediation of the process. It is wrong to derive educational objectives from subject content, especially when there must be a temptation on the part of the practitioner-turned-teacher to put more and more subject matter into the curriculum with, in addition to the proliferation noted above, the further tendency to indulge in rigid subject compartmentalisation and to reduce all educational objectives to low-level knowledge-based objectives, such as '1.2 — recalling facts', because of pressure of time, while many more valuable educational activities are neglected. Relationships and principles are more vital than facts; applying, and being influenced by what is learned is even more vital than memorising it. The student should not learn the subject matter: she should learn *from* subject matter.

Nevertheless, even though the subject content be only a vehicle for learning, it is important that the vehicle should be appropriate for its work and well-maintained. The question of its appropriateness has been settled already by the discipline of the task analysis and the resulting list of tasks, but this is the time to ensure that all the elements of subject content necessary to the execution of the nursing tasks concerned have been added to a Summary Tabulation of the curriculum and its educational objectives in something like the manner shown in Table 11.1. If preferred, this allocation of subject content could be done as each educational objective is constructed initially, but the device of completing the objectives, tabulating them and then adding subject content and other items to the tabulation tends to keep the work moving along fairly briskly and helps to keep things more clearly in perspective and in balance.

On completion of this work the designer should then go through the whole sequence of educational objectives, changes sought, educational skills and exercises recommended and the subject content recommended, checking every aspect with particular reference to filling any gaps in the subject content provision (an unlikely eventuality if the proper procedures are followed) and to eliminating any unnecessary duplication of content. In connection with this latter concern it should be pointed out again that you will find that a certain amount of repetition ('redundancy') can be extremely valuable in reinforcing and widening pre-existent knowledge by presenting it again at new levels and in new contexts. This will become more apparent in the next section of the present Step and you may well find yourself actually seeking opportunities to build in redundancy quite deliberately for these purposes.

The arrangement and organisation of the curriculum content

The next step is the arrangement and organisation of the educational objective packages of learning experiences and subject matter. These features of the course are oriented towards and shaped by the purposes of the teachers, based upon the foundations of the philosophy, model and list of tasks. Further than this, it is only feasible to proceed on the strength of hypotheses as to the kind of arrangement and organisation which should, all else being equal, give the desired outcomes within the constraints set by the

Table 11.1 Sample curriculum summary tabulation: Part 1.

Overall aim: Section 11 of the 'List of Nursing Tasks': 'Practical implementation of nursing care techniques'
Subsidiary goal: Section 11 Sub-section 5 of the 'List of Nursing Tasks': 'Deal with problems in … infection … preparation for and carrying out of procedures …'

Educational objectives	Changes sought	Educational skills and exercises	Subject content
11.5.17.1 Aseptic dressing technique: Preamble			
(a) Circumstances in which dressings are done (b) Roles of the nurse (c) Aseptic dressings: problems research i.e. criteria and circumstances for:	Orientation to a set-piece task with responsibility for a patient	K1.1 – 1.10 2.1 – 2.2 A1.1 – 1.2 3.3	Revise healing of wounds; function and nature of dressings; revise the autonomy of patient; revise roles of the nurse; nature of infection; problems of control and principles of asepsis
11.5.17.2 Aseptic dressing technique: Preparation			
(a) Hazards and counter-measures (b) Preparation of patient (c) Preparation of trolley (d) Preparation of self i.e. rehearsal for:	Awareness of need for care in preparation and execution of tasks	K1.4 – 1.8 A3.1 S2	Transmission of infection, especially human role; defences against transmission of infection; revise counselling; revise lifting and moving patients; contents and layout of trolley; revise personal hygiene; preparation of self for aseptic procedures
11.5.17.3 Aseptic dressing technique: Execution			
(a) Brief assistant (b) Place trolley (c) Place and reassure patient (d) Inspect and cleanse wound (e) Apply dressing (f) Return patient to ward and counsel (g) Dispose of equipment and supplies (h) Complete records and reports	Leadership; attitude of caring; psychomotor skills; coherence in written and verbal records and presentations	K1.1 – 1.10 2.1 – 2.2 3; 4; 5.1 – 5.2 A1.1 – 1.3 2.3; 3.3; 4.1 S2; 3; 4.1; 4.2; 5.1	Flow-charting as means of communication; skills of removing and replacing dressings in aseptic conditions; clean/infected wounds and implications for patient; disposal of infected items; documentation and reporting

Refer to schedule of educational objectives (Step 7) for full details and see page 154 for Part 2.

institution, and which can be tested in practice and, if necessary, modified. It must not be forgotten that the initial choice and any subsequent modification of the philosophical, task-based and subject content elements will determine to a large extent the organisation and administration of the course and the methods of learning, teaching and assessing and that any changes on one side of this equation must be matched by appropriate changes on the other side.

There are a number of modes of organising a course such as this:

1. There is no reason why the curriculum should not follow the order of elements as laid down in the philosophy starting with the study of the client and his familial and social background and proceeding through areas concerned with health and the nurse's role before reaching the theory, functions and activities of nursing and the considerations of nursing law and ethics and professional matters. This order is also reflected in the model and in the list of tasks and would therefore appear to be a natural choice for the order of the course.

    You should, however, be aware of one or two problems associated with this *subject-led approach*. One is that there might be a natural tendency to set up and maintain, however inadvertently, narrow, distinct and mutually exclusive subject compartments in the arrangement of the course, possibly even administered and taught by distinct and mutually exclusive subject-based departments or teams within the school. As an extreme case, it might even happen that nursing might follow the example of some other vocational studies, housed in universities and polytechnics, which, instead of designating a skeleton of nursing subjects which might quite reasonably include elements of science, sociology and psychology, would actually assume an exoskeleton by studying nursing *within* the context of one of these alien subject-disciplines thus being irrevocably distorted as far as that institution was concerned.

    It would also create a tendency, as has been already suggested, for very specific subjects to be crowded into the curriculum on very dubious grounds in some cases and taught rather superficially to relatively low-level, knowledge-based objectives in the area of the mere 'recall of facts' because of shortage of time and resources to offer a more effective and beneficial treatment of the material. This would be quite unacceptable, in spite of the ready repertoires of factual knowledge and the articulate, if limited 'thinking' that might be demonstrated in the aftermath. It is widely believed that the subject-based arrangement is not suitable for students coming fresh to the course or beginning work in a sector that is strange to them and who are not yet ready for self-instructional techniques or other learning methods which require a greater than normal degree of responsibility for their own progress.

2. The *needs approach* is the most free and flexible approach to arranging and organising a curriculum since, in this case, the curriculum is intended to be responsive to the students' needs of the moment and, in fact, to have virtually no arrangement or organisation except in so far as it follows these needs as they emerge and are identified. This ensures that the curriculum is in a constant state of flux or rolling change and is therefore likely to be neither useful for guidance nor popular.

3. The *activity curriculum* is of interest in being based almost entirely upon a sequence of activities or interests but although it is relatively unplanned it is not necessarily intended to reflect the needs of the students in the form in which the students see them.

4. The *broad-field curriculum* lies somewhere between these extremes in that narrow subject-specialisms are replaced by a broader structure which nevertheless remains firm. It is based upon the broad operational areas of health care such as those noted under paragraph 1 above as being the main elements of the philosophy and model, but without unduly slavish adherence to the normal divisions of the list of tasks. There is much to be commended here in the integration and enrichment of knowledge and skills over areas of related, theme-based studies and the promotion of attitudes, which seldom, if ever, involve allegiance to narrow specialisms.

5. The *core curriculum* is much more complex than just a collection of the important or central subjects or topics, as is usually thought to be the case. In relation to the arrangement and organisation of the curriculum, a number of intentions on the part of the designer may be combined to form a pattern. They may be correlated to illuminate and promote a number of themes drawn from aspects of life in general or from the particular field of nursing, from its current issues and problems and from the carefully identified and negotiated needs of the general body of students, as opposed to the needs of a particular intake on a particular day. It is important that these matters, whatever their nature and origins, should be such as are likely to provide appropriate inspiration and substance for learning and, over a period of time, combine to produce a solid and comprehensive foundation of the principles and practices that are common to nurses everywhere and without which they cannot claim to be 'nurses' in any real sense.

You might, in fact, come to the conclusion that virtually the whole programme is of such universal significance that you are reluctant to designate any parts as 'core' or 'not core' and it is perfectly reasonable to declare an 'all-core' or 'no-core' curriculum. It amounts to the same thing! In these circumstances much learning and teaching can be done by problem-solving and other investigatory means with a wide variety of learning and teaching methods, in flexibly timetabled units, and possibly with a rather greater degree of planning by, and guidance of, the students than is commonly the case. There are no firm divisions between the subjects that are permitted to be covered, but therein lies the opportunity for relatively untrammelled planning round the educational objectives, and their influence upon the students, that are the keys to the curriculum design process. The danger, as before, is the difficulty of avoiding excessive compartmentalisation of study on the one hand and unacceptable diffuseness on the other.

The core curriculum approach is a sound way of dealing with the problem of preparing the students during their basic education to make the best use of opportunities in post-basic education which will demand a much more mature attitude to the process of learning. Basic principles, once learned, can be applied to any other context where they are relevant if the student has the time and the ability to transfer knowledge efficiently.

All or any of these modes of arranging and organising the educational objectives packages of the curriculum and the course, may be used singly or simultaneously in different parts of a curriculum as and when it seems appropriate to do so. They are not mutually exclusive. In particular, the structuring of studies in a continuous flow should enable work to be planned in a smooth progression without conflicts of interest, bottle-necks, or periodical over-loading of students with ill-timed essays and projects from a variety of uncoordinated sources. It also ensures that all the work being done in the main programme at any one time is directly relevant to the current basic theme, if there is one, and it permits experiences and content to be realistically weighted by, for example, time units of one teaching period each or by some other criterion, in accordance with the intrinsic importance and desirable depth of study of each part of the topic, regardless of any arbitrary concept of 'core' or 'non-core' or any other special status.

It might be useful to turn for a moment to the consideration of some major divisions of the curriculum which might be created for specific functions concerned with the status of the students rather than with that of the subject matter.

1. An *induction course* may be employed as a preliminary taster for the whole programme. Some of its more academic elements may be designed to familiarise the intending nurse with the nature, potential and probable flavour of nursing in broad outline. These could be presented at the level of knowing and of comprehending, in easily-assimilated audio-visual formats for the most part. Other induction course elements may be intended for a variety of purposes such as getting to know the layout and personalities of the school and of the hospitals of the district, familiarisation with the

facilities, especially with library and domestic provision, and, perhaps, the beginnings of getting to know each other on some outdoor exercise or other event. The student could be regarded as free to leave at any time during the two weeks or so of the duration of this course with a minimum of disruption and waste of time for all concerned although there should be time for adequate discussion and counselling in this matter for any who remained doubtful or uncommitted.

2. A *foundation course* should be regarded as an integral part of the 'spiral curriculum', unlike the induction course, but it, too, might profitably be informative rather than analytical, confined to topics selected from what would be your 'common core' if you were to have one in the main programme.

3. The question of *optional* or *elective* studies (you will find both of these terms in use for the one concept) is a more open decision. Even if it is desired to create a range of studies to suit students' interests in areas of non-core, non-essential subject matter, these can only be arranged in a particular institution in the light of the experience, interests and abilities of the members of the teaching staff, the facilities available in the school and the locality, the topics which are of some concern to the profession at the time, and the wishes of the students as expressed by their uptake of the studies on offer. Such studies need not be confined to nursing proper but might be intended to cater for the sociology which might be sought by students concerned to work in the community, or the background biological sciences or the practical, educational aspects of health education work. Perhaps one afternoon each week might be devoted to such studies with one optional study to be undertaken each year, supporting main-stream teaching where possible and being taught and assessed to the same standard.

4. A *revision course* is self explanatory and something of a luxury, being substantially tailor-made for the needs of individual students and representing a particularly heavy commitment of staff time and effort.

The sequence of learning

The choice of the sequence of learning within whatever broad arrangement and organisation is adopted tends to be somewhat arbitrary, although the purposes of a given piece of learning must be allowed to dictate the timing as well as the form and nature of the session where this is feasible. Various principles may be employed. The chronological or evolutionary development of a subject is a clear enough guide but is hardly exciting and could be stultifying: the logical structure of a subject has already been advocated as suitable for the broader arrangement and organisation of the course as long as the students are aware of, and fully appreciate, the significance of that structure: a progression from simple to more complex concepts may help:

likewise, a progression from principles to practical applications might be appropriate in some circumstances, although it is hard to imagine a learner-driver enduring six weeks of lectures before actually entering a vehicle other than as a passenger.

Alternative sequences that might be considered according to their relevance include the opposite trend, from concrete practice to abstract principles; from familiar concepts into the unknown; from easy to more difficult learning. The selection of a sequence – and again, a number may be used singly or simultaneously in different parts of the curriculum – is often settled by the answer to the eminently practical question: 'What is it necessary to know or feel or experience before starting to learn "x"?' This may be tackled empirically, but in nursing, as in some other vocational studies, the teacher is often fortunate enough to be the subject expert and practitioner as well as the teacher, rather than being subject to second-hand advice from an outside authority on how to arrange and sequence a course.

The decision as to whether or not to adopt the *spiral curriculum* style of sequence for a complex course scheduled to last for several years is now almost a foregone conclusion in favour of sequencing certain kinds and levels of learning to cumulate in relatively small units at different points in, say, a three-year period, in order to keep pace with the unfolding of the overall subject of nursing and with the students' growing awareness and maturity in professional terms. This is a matter for commonsense consideration and would probably be done in any case without a formal decision or special terminology. It means that important parts of the subject are re-visited from time to time in different contexts, viewed from different aspects, appreciated at different levels of complexity and assessed in different ways. Successive visits will feature variations in the precision of knowledge; balance of concepts; range of facts, comparisons and relations defined; and the kind of applications made or suggested – all with an increasing tendency towards greater complexity and abstraction as time goes on.

The disadvantages are slight and the problem of this 'splintering' of a subject, as it might be termed by its detractors, is of little significance if skilfully done with the students' benefit in mind. Of course, if the educational loss is prohibitive you should not splinter that topic; do not even spiral at all if you foresee no clear benefit in doing so. If you *do* wish to consider this more closely, there is a diagram which might help in the 'Brief outline' chapter of this book.

A rather similar mode of manipulating the elements of a course is represented by the concept of *alternative samples of content*. The principle is that different individuals or groups of students may be allocated to study different parts or aspects of a topic simultaneously, according to their own particular interests. For example, this is a very effective way in which to engage the interest of overseas students who contemplate returning home to practise and teach, or other similar groups with special concerns not normally considered in the ordinary course of events to require special treatment. This is already a familiar ploy in primary and secondary schools but in vocational education might be less effective because students at this level, with a career at stake, often exhibit something akin to panic if they find that fellow-students in another group are learning subject content which has apparently been 'omitted' from their own work schedule. This sort of happening tends to create the very kind of bewilderment which the curriculum design process and consultation are intended to minimise. There is also the problem that, if the object is to equip every student comprehensively with the proverbial bird's-eye view of the subject, there will inevitably be gaps in the learning of some members of a course, however well-organised the inter-group follow-up discussions and feedback might be.

At this stage the curriculum is probably in the form of a carefully-considered and appropriate sequence of packages, each comprising one or more educational objectives with their prescriptions for change of student outlook or behaviour and the necessary educational exercises and subject content, as demonstrated in the tabulation reproduced earlier in this Step.

The sequence will have been determined by:

1. The course to which the packages contribute: Induction, Foundation, Main core, Main non-core, Option or Revision course element and then, within each course by–
2. Major areas of study to which the packages contribute, sub-divided by subjects and subsidiary topics, with different parts probably dispersed to various levels of the curriculum spiral or, alternatively, left in order as a 'straight-through' sequence from start to finish, according to the decision of the curriculum team.

The curriculum as thus presented is intended to be appropriate to the requirements of the supervisory board, the needs of the students, the needs of the local and national service sectors and the local resources available to the teachers.

Derivation of lesson units

It is now a suitable juncture at which to draw breath before going on to:

1. Break down the chain of educational objective packages and their subject content into individual lesson units to fit the lesson periods which are the norm at your particular school or department. These are conventionally of about fifty minutes' duration but if they could be made more flexible than this, teaching and learning would benefit enormously. This is, in effect, a weighting system for topics.

2. Determine at what points the course should be divided into modules, academic terms, school-based blocks and any other administrative, as opposed to educational, constraints that are imposed upon the flow of learning and teaching.

The individual lesson units may be regarded as *focusing centres* (another term which you may come across in curriculum design literature), each one based upon some phenomenon such as a concept and a relevant book chapter, a journal article, a video-tape, a discussion, simulation, formal lecture or visit – anything, in fact, which may be used to trigger off a piece of learning which contributes to the achievement of an educational objective. Each such focusing centre, broad or narrow, is both a key element in its own right and a link with something else in the curriculum, another focusing centre, with which a connection, once made, will evoke mutual, two-way illumination for the promotion of understanding, feeling and skill by means of a fresh and challenging association and reinforcement that would not otherwise have existed. You should begin to identify and make these links now.

It is also an appropriate stage at which to sit down once more with your Tabulation of Educational Objectives and their associated data and check, as far as possible, that the course does hang together as a unitary whole in spite of the many separate educational units and administrative divisions for which allowance must be made; that the specified subject content is likely to contribute to the success of the educational exercises in assisting the students to achieve each educational objective and bring about the desired changes within themselves; and that these changes lie within the specification and the spirit of the nursing philosophy and model which you adopted. This is a major check on the nearly-completed curriculum and serves also as a 'dry-run' for the main 'validation' in the next Step.

Incidentally, in view of all this checking and possible changing of the details of the curriculum that might result, you might consider, now that it is almost complete, whether or not to mount the whole proposal upon a computer in order to:

1. Create a permanent, compact but adjustable record.
2. Experiment with the many variations on this basic configuration which will no doubt suggest themselves to various members of the team and of the wider circle of people consulted up to this point.
3. Experiment with subsequent modifications that will be indicated by the validation and evaluation processes yet to come in the next Step and beyond.
4. Comply with any requirements of the supervisory board which have not yet been promulgated.
5. Review the whole curriculum at regular intervals during its working life.

The forging of links

This matter of the making of links across the length and breadth of the curriculum has already received a brief mention but it now requires serious consideration before any further progress is made in finalising the curriculum and while there is still an opportunity to apply particular methods of learning, teaching and assessing to the topics concerned so as to emphasise their essential unity or relationships. These topics may be identical in some important respect, similar or complementary, occurring in different contexts and levels of the course, as for example, in the spiral formation which is designed to show up these relationships. These links should be noted in your copy of the curriculum tabulation and the links made or confirmed.

A backward look in particular, can be most valuable as a means of reinforcing and revising material, but the main value of the linking suggested is as a way of stressing the essential unity and integration of the curriculum. While not of itself a vital element, this air of being self-contained and self-sufficient nevertheless helps to foster confidence in the product on the part of those teachers, students and others in whose working lives the curriculum is a central feature.

The allocation of learning and teaching methods

Russell and Latcham have neatly and succinctly summed up the curriculum designer's dilemma in this matter:

> What kinds of learning situation are there? The variety is endless as skilful teachers will vary their techniques according to their immediate perceptions of the situations that their students are encountering . . . we may classify simultaneously by the way the students are organised, by the media used, by the activities of the students and by the structuring of the learning or subject material . . . we also recognise that, with the feedback received, teachers will make appropriate adjustments and variations in the methods used.[1]

In this quotation the concept of the rapid adjustment of learning and teaching modes by teachers who are sensitive to feedback from their students occurs twice in a short paragraph only thirteen lines long, even in its original form, and the concept of 'variety' or 'variation' occurs three times. Several ways of regarding learning and teaching methods are suggested. It would seem to be of little use, therefore, to list extensively and to describe in detail all conceivable methods of learning and teaching: in any case, this has been done already with much greater expertise than could be summoned up here in a wide range of easily accessible publications, of which a selection is offered in the list of further reading appended to this Step.

Nor is it considered appropriate to make firm recommendations for the learning and teaching methods to be adopted for each lesson unit, although specimen suggestions are made later in this Step (Table 11.2) as an example of how such recommendations could be presented in a curriculum tabulation (this is Part 2 of the tabulation of which Part 1, dealing with objectives and subject content, was presented earlier in this Step in Table 11.1).

Much must be left to local autonomy and to the judgement of the teachers in each school or department, partly as a mark of respect for their ability to prescribe for their own local circumstances, talents, preferences, funds and facilities, partly because of the need, acknowledged above, to leave them free to react to feedback from their own particular groups of students, and partly because the outline learning and teaching methods of many of the lesson units are already expressed or implied in the relevant tabulations as, for example, 'library-based investigation'; 'demonstration in role-play'; 'completion of a fictitious set of records' and so on. It may, however, be useful to close this section with a glance at a classification of learning and teaching methods which is based in part upon the opening quotation above, in order that you may be reminded, if that were necessary, of the major parameters involved in making recommendations of your own. The initial division is a dichotomy between:

1. Direct experience of the subject matter or process for students by means of visits, simulations, surveys, clinical experience periods and so on.
2. Vicarious experience largely synonymous with second-hand, but quite possibly very appropriate and effective, techniques of a conventional 'class-room' nature: lectures, readings, viewings, listenings, self-instruction, discussions *about* the topic.

A set of subdivisions common to each of these two major categories of learning and teaching methods and suggested by the quotation above, might comprise:

1. The organisation of students and teachers as defined by:
   (a) The size of the group(s).
   (b) The adoption of individual pacing or corporate progression.
   (c) The timing of study – in fixed short periods or more flexible patterns.
   (d) The frequency of meetings – weekly, daily or almost continuous on demand.
   (e) The intervals betwen learning and feedback.
   (f) The method of working – the group in unison, 'alternative samples' worked by sub-groups or individuals, individual projects, and so on.
   (g) Deployment of teachers – singly or in pairs or teams.
2. The media in use:
   (a) Books and journals.
   (b) Structured self-instructional materials.

    (c) Still visual aids.
    (d) Film, videotape, live television off-air.
    (e) Sound recordings and radio off-air.
    (f) Realia, models and simulations.
3. The activities of the students: knowing and comprehending:
    (a) Listening to live exposition.
    (b) Reading, listening to or viewing processed expository items.
    (c) Working individually through structured learning materials.
    (d) Investigating and discovering in real-life situations.
    (e) Making notes.
    (f) Forming concepts.
4. The activities of students: showing competence:
    (a) Constructing and applying – in real-life situations.
    (b) Constructing and applying – in simulated situations.
5. The activities of students: showing understanding:
    (a) Analysing and synthesising reports and plans.
    (b) Testing and evaluating plans and recommendations.
6. The activities of students: being changed by experiences:
    (a) Thinking creatively.
    (b) Presenting and discussing reports.
    (c) Interacting in the exercise of social skills.
    (d) Receiving, responding to, valuing, organising and adopting values and expressing these as attitudes.
7. Structuring materials into lesson units:
    (a) Selecting an appropriate mode of integrating learning exercises and subject content into lesson units by evolutionary, concrete-to-abstract, familiar-to-unfamiliar or other principles.
    (b) Creating a spiral structure of Induction, Foundation, Main core, Main non-core, Options, Revision and other types of course elements.
    (c) Creating remedial loops for the needs of students: an obvious use for the 'alternative samples' technique.
    (d) Making progress by the 'straight-line' addition of small increments of learning.
    (e) Making progress by large and apparently random steps, subject to a concluding 'round-up'.
    (f) Leaving students to reach their own conclusions under some mutually acceptable degree of guidance.
    (g) Reacting to feedback from the students once they have been briefed, but taking no other initiative on their behalf.

Table 11.2 Sample curriculum summary tabulation: Part 2.

Objective designation	Lesson units and lesson weighting in 55 min. units	Direct or vicarious	Learning/teaching method and timing	Assessment method and standard	Links to other lesson units
11.5.17.1	*Aseptic dressing technique:* *Preamble* (a) Circumstances in which dressings done 1 (b) Roles of nurse (c) Aseptic dressings: problems research	V	Library investigation 30 discussion 10 Written report 15	Formal assessment of written work x	5.1; 5.2; care 11.5; 16.2 dressings
11.5.17.2	*Aseptic dressing technique:* *Preparation* (a) Hazards and counter-measures 1 (b) Preparation of patient (c) Preparation of trolley (d) Preparation of self	D live simulation	Draws diagram 10 Guided Demonstration followed by non-guided demonstration by student 30	Formal assessment of diagram x Graded 0 – 5 5	11.4; 11.3; 11.5; 16.2; 12.1.5
11.5.17.3	*Aseptic dressing technique:* *Execution* (a) Brief assistant (b) Place trolley (c) Place and reassure patient (d) Inspect and cleanse wound *dresser and assistant change roles* 2 (e) apply dressing (f) return patient to ward and counsel (g) dispose of equipment and supplies (h) complete records and reports	V D live simulation V	Flow-chart 10 demonstration by tutor 25 Guided demonstration by students in pairs 30 Non-guided demonstration by volunteer pair 30 Exposition by tutor 10	Formal assessment of flow chart x	13.2.2 11.4; 11.5; 16.2; 12.1.5 10.4

Note: This sheet would normally be attached end-on to Sample Curriculum Summary Sheet Part 1 (see page 143) in order to form a tabulation spread-sheet.

Allocation of methods of assessment

Again, it is not the purpose of this book to present a comprehensive survey and comparative critical study of methods of assessing the performance of students. In so far as our students are being prepared for a formal qualification, awarded at the ultimate discretion of a professional body, it must be accepted that the expressed wishes of that body in this matter must be respected and its specification maintained in the final, and perhaps certain interim assessments, even under a regime of internal assessment.

However, assessment at other levels and at other interim points in the course may still be arranged by the local school or department and at the lowest levels, if no other, by the teacher. Such assessment must therefore find a place on your Tabulation of educational objectives, exercises, subject content and learning/teaching methods, specimen pages of which are reproduced in this Step. The primary purpose of assessment is not the establishment of a competitive rank order of students in a group or school, nor the perpetuation of a subtle form of social control; neither is it an arcane academic ritual. It is required only to ascertain whether or not the student has achieved the educational objectives and become characterised by the changes which the objectives were designed to produce in her. Of course, this anticipates the substance of Steps 9 and 10 which require the curriculum designer to prove beyond all reasonable doubt that the curriculum *is* capable of producing those changes in a nominally successful student and that it can go on doing that for successive generations of students in that institution and for similar groups of students elsewhere.

This purpose requires only that a student can be shown to have achieved, or failed to achieve, a satisfactory score or performance at the time of assessment. Elaborate percentages, grades and awards of honours and distinctions should, strictly speaking, be quite irrelevant to the purpose and it is a moot point whether or not they should ever be published or used except as confidential data for the internal use of the profession, and then, presumably, only to the advantage of the student. Even in the extreme case of operant conditioning, it is the fact of 'success', rather than the degree of success, that provides adequate reward, or motivation as the case may be, for the subject who is not to be encouraged to either bask upon her laurels or sulk behind them, but to get up and get on with the next indicated phase of learning, whether that be advance or revision.

For the teachers, short-term assessment of students should be regarded intrinsically as feedback, reflecting upon their own teaching ability, methods, facilities, resources and, indeed, assessment methods themselves. When correlated with what is known of the students in their academic and practical activities, this feedback should inform teachers of the extent to which their aims, goals and objectives are being achieved, the likely reasons for non-achievement and the changes which they, the teachers, should make to improve the performance of their students. It also enables them to infuence the behaviour of students in a positive way – to make them work harder generally or more selectively in a specialised area – inducing some useful degree of concern or pressure but naturally stopping short of creating anxiety or depression.

The difficulty lies in yet another sphere: the attempt to use assessments as a means of predicting the student's future fitness to practise as a professional in real-life situations over a working lifetime of up to forty years or more. This difficulty occurs at two points in the period of education: the pre-entry selection, when even whole batteries of tests, formally administered by members of the British Psychological Society may not resolve queries about a student's general or specialised abilities, and also at the assessment which leads directly to the final qualification to practise professionally. It may be useful at this point to sketch a brief classification of assessment methods in order that you, the curriculum designer, may be assisted to recall the options available for discussion with your teacher-colleagues. These options are listed under six category headings:

1. Phase of the course:
     (a) Pre-entry testing.
     (b) Entry tests.
     (c) Interim (e.g. annual) assessments.
     (d) End of course assessments.
     (e) Continuous assessment.
     (f) Assessment after a stipulated period of in-post service.
2. Student activity:
     (a) Writing answers in essay form.
     (b) Minimal response answers – for example, ticking multiple-choice question boxes.
     (c) Oral (viva voce) discussion.
     (d) Practical task performance.
3. Type of test:
     (a) Short essay.
     (b) Multiple-choice question test.
     (c) Thesis, dissertation, long essay, major project report.
     (d) Practical task or extended clinical practice.
     (e) Continuous course-work assessment.
     (f) Attitude-assessment by non-cognitive tests.
     (g) Impressionistic, 'intuitive', assessment.
4. Conditions under which assessment takes place:
     (a) Unseen examination.
     (b) Open-book examination.

    (c) Pre-published questions.
    (d) Pre-published course marks with option to redeem failure or enhance marginal success by taking a formal assessment.
    (e) Self-assessment by subjective profiling.
    (f) Peer-group assessment by fellow students.
5. Duration of assessment:
    (a) Conventional three-hour paper.
    (b) Flexible but not unlimited duration.
    (c) Short tests, e.g. 15 minutes, cumulated over a given period.
    (d) Extended, long-term test, e.g. thesis as in 3(c) above.

When dealing with your colleagues, the following comments about commonly held assumptions regarding assessment methods might be borne in mind:

1. Examinations appear to be designed to repress rather than to promote the special qualities of mind which they are sometimes assumed to highlight: originality, critical thinking, and organising ability.
2. Capacities of a practical nature are seldom adequately assessed although certain kinds of tests are assumed to do this: these abilities are vital to many professional workers, including nurses, and weigh heavily with potential employers.
3. Since an examination is assumed to put a student in a 'real-life' situation, albeit on paper, it is assumed in some quarters that it should therefore be stressful and competitive; although students commonly suffer from depressive illnesses and hysteria and even attempt suicide in significant numbers, the examination rarely requires more than theoretical knowledge and the ability to write short essays in reasonable English.
4. Oddly enough, in spite of the often-encountered desire to test students under 'real-life' conditions, they are normally examined as isolated individuals, separated from their colleagues with whom they have studied and worked, and separated by a temporary barrier of professional impersonality from the teacher who has taught, counselled and led them.
5. It is usually assumed that a Gaussian or 'bell-shaped' curve of normal distribution, which commonly results from the plotting of assessment scores, is an essential instrument of control. Institutions blame the examination alike for a big crop of either very good or very poor results and attempt to re-jig the examination system to 'restore' the desired curve; they seldom rejoice with their students at mass success or blame themselves for mass failure.
6. Examinations are almost invariably placed at the end of the course where every winning post is expected to be. This tends to distract students and rob the outcome of its true significance as students approach the

beginning of their life-work in the practice of their profession. There are better ways of timing assessment as has been suggested above. Even continuous assessment methods may not be free from this, or indeed, some of the other constraints mentioned here.

7. As has already been indicated, there is little justification for the assumption that the outside world needs a detailed verdict on each student. Anyone who has been selected with some care in the first place and has achieved 'success' in a well-taught course based upon a well-organised curriculum should make a perfectly adequate nurse and would speedily reveal any outstanding abilities or minor weaknesses in clinical practice.

Useful criteria for a scheme of assessment should, perhaps, include the following:

1. It should enhance, rather than detract from, the efficacy and pleasure of learning and teaching.
2. It should not place an undue burden on the time, effort and well-being of students and teachers in completing, administering and marking whatever type of assessment is adopted, neither should the aftermath be any more distressing than is absolutely necessary for the unfortunate ones.
3. It must be valid – that is, it must measure, as accurately as is desired, what it is designed to measure. This is one of the reasons why curriculum objectives, exercises and subject content must be clearly and systematically constructed rather than merely 'put together' on an *ad hoc* basis, since they are the given data of the assessment procedure.
4. Assessment must also be reliable as between individual students of a given group and, over a period of time, between successive generations of student groups; it must also be reliable in producing similar results in other institutions with comparable students and teachers working on comparable courses.

These are only broad observations about assessment in general for the benefit of the curriculum designer. The list of further reading will lead you to books and articles dealing in greater detail with the pros and cons of particular methods of assessment in nursing and, of course, these are only a selection from the available material.

References

1. Further Education Staff College, *Curriculum development in further education: papers* by John Russell and Jack Latcham, Coombe Lodge, Blagdon, Further Education Staff College, 1979.

Further reading

ARRANGEMENT AND ORGANISATION OF THE CURRICULUM
Sugden, John, Model education, *Senior Nurse*, 15 August 1984, Vol. 1, No. 20, pp. 10–13. ('My model was constructed as a three-dimensional representation of [five] specific themes... in a deliberate quantitative and spatial relationship to each other and which were relative [to each other] on a chronological basis'.)

LEARNING AND TEACHING METHODS: A SELECTION
Allen, Hazel, O., Murrell, John (editors), *Nurse training: an enterprise in curriculum development at St Thomas' Hospital*, Plymouth, Macdonald and Evans, 1978, Chs. 5 and 6.
Beard, Ruth M., *Research into teaching methods in higher education, mainly in British universities*, 2nd edn, London, Society for Research into Higher Education Ltd, 1968.
Beard, Ruth M., Hartley, James, *Teaching and learning in higher education*, 4th edn, London, Harper & Row, 1984.
Burnard, Philip, The teacher as facilitator, *Senior Nurse*, June 1985, Vol. 3, No. 1, pp. 34–37. (Note: his reference no. 16 should read: *Nursing Mirror*, 2 March 1983, Vol. 156, No. 9, pp. 29–34.)
Burnard, Philip, Playing the game in nurse education (role play), *Nursing Times*, 1 April 1987, Vol. 83, No. 13, pp. 61–63.
Butler, Barbara, Elliott, Doreen, *Teaching and learning for practice (social work)*, Aldershot, Gower, 1985, Chs. 2–6.
Curzon, L.B., *Teaching in further education: an outline of principles and practice*, London, Cassell, 1976.
Greaves, Fred, Learning the scientific method (the problem-solving approach), *Senior Nurse*, June 1987, Vol. 6, No. 6, pp. 23–24.
Gwinnett, Anne, Massie, S., Integrating computers into the curriculum: a development project, *Nurse Education Today*, June 1986, Vol. 6, No. 3, pp. 129–132.
Hancock, Paula K, Making the most of the media (A/V), *Nurse Education Today*, June 1986, Vol. 6, No. 3, pp. 124–128.
Hinchliff, Susan M. (editor) *Teaching clinical nursing*, 2nd edn, Edinburgh, Churchill Livingstone, 1986.
Jarvis, Peter, Contract learning *Journal of District Nursing*, November 1986, Vol. 5, No. 6, pp. 13–14.
Jarvis, Peter, *Professional education*, London, Croom Helm, 1983, Ch. 6.
Jarvis, Peter, Gibson, Sheila, *The teacher practitioner in nursing, midwifery and health visiting*, London, Croom Helm, 1985, Ch. 2–5.
Kilty, James, *Experiential learning*, Guildford, Human Potential Research Project, Department of Educational Studies, University of Surrey, 1986. ('... aims to demystify the term 'experiential learning' without glossing over its subtleties... [so that] teachers of nursing may help learners to gain more from their practical experience'.)
Marson, S.N., Ward sister – teacher or facilitator? An investigation into the behavioural characteristics of effective ward teachers, *Journal of Advanced Nursing*, 1982, July Vol. 7, No. 4, pp. 347–357.

Nursing Times and Distance Learning Centre, South Bank Polytechnic, Teaching nurses: 3 supplements, *Nursing Times*, 1986, Vol. 82, Nos. 16, 21 and 24.

Raichura, Liz, Learning by doing, *Nursing Times*, 1 April 1987, Vol. 83, No. 13, pp. 59–61.

Sellek, Thelma, Variation on a theme, *Nursing Mirror*, 19 August 1981, Vol. 153, No. 8, pp. 30–31 (Group and individual learning with a central theme of problem-solving).

ASSESSMENT METHODS: A SELECTION

Beard, Ruth M., Hartley, James, *Teaching and learning in higher education*, 4th edn, London, Harper & Row, 1984, Ch. 14, Evaluating students, courses and teachers.

Butler, Barbara, Elliott, Doreen, *Teaching and learning for practice*, Aldershot, Gower, 1985, Ch. 7.

Castledine, George, Assessing ward assessments, *Nursing Mirror*, 5 April 1979, Vol. 148, No. 14, p. 10).

Curzon, L.B., *Teaching in further education: an outline of principles and practice*, London, Cassell, 1976, Chs. XVI and XVII.

Frisbie, David, A., Testing achievement beyond the knowledge level, *Journal of Nursing Education*, 1983, Vol. 22, No. 6, pp. 228–231.

Heron, John, *Assessment*, London, British Postgraduate Medical Federation, University of London and Human Potential Research Project, Department of Adult Education, University of Surrey, 1981.

Heywood, John, *Assessment in higher education*, Chichester, Wiley, 1977.

Hinchliff, Susan M. (editor), *Teaching clinical nursing*, 2nd edn, Edinburgh, Churchill Livingstone, 1986.

Jarvis, Peter, *Professional education*, London, Croom Helm, 1983, Ch. 7, Appraisal in professional education.

Jarvis, Peter, Gibson, Sheila, *The teacher practitioner in nursing, midwifery and health visiting*, London, Croom Helm, 1985, Ch. 6, Assessing students.

Jefferies, P.M., Tibbles, H.J., Continuous assessment within the King's Health District, *Nursing Times*, 21 August 1980, Vol. 76, No. 34, Occasional papers, Vol. 76, No. 20, pp. 89–92.

Kilty, James, *Self and peer assessment and peer audit: paper given at the Annual Conference of the Society for Research into Higher Education, Brighton, December 1979*, Guildford, Human Potential Research Project, Department of Educational Studies, University of Surrey, 1979.

Kehoe, Derek M., Harker, Tom, *Principles of assessing nursing skills*, London, Pitman Medical, 1979.

King's Fund Hospital Centre and General Nursing Council Working Party *Assessment: a guide for the completion of progress reports on nurses in training*, London, King Edward's Hospital Fund for London, 1972.

Law, Bill, *Uses and abuses of profiling: a handbook on reviewing and recording student experience and achievement*, London, Harper & Row, 1984.

Nursing Times and Distance Learning Centre, South Bank Polytechnic, Assessing nurses: 3 supplements, *Nursing Times*, 1986, Vol. 82, Nos. 31, 35 and 39.

Sellek, Thelma, The future of assessment, *Nursing Mirror*, 4 August 1982, Vol. 155, No. 5, Education forum supplement No. 5, pp. vii–viii.
Sheehan, John, Assessing learning: continuous assessment versus final examinations, *Nurse Education Today*, April 1985, Vol. 5, No. 2, pp. 49–55.
Young, Ann P., Morgan, Wendy, Continuous assessment for nurses in the Thomas Guy School of Nursing, *Nursing Times*, 21/28 December 1978 and 4 January 1979, Vol. 74, No. 51, and Vol. 75, No. 1, Occasional papers, Vol. 74, No. 35, pp. 141–144 and Vol. 75, No. 1, pp. 1–3.

Chapter 12

Step 9 Reviewing, presenting and implementing the completed curriculum

Reminder

Validation is the process of determining, as far as you can, whether or not the newly-completed curriculum is likely to be able to do in practice whatever you designed it to do. Presentation of the curriculum is akin to the printing and publication of a book, with a number of external requirements to be accommodated. Even implementation is not the last word – hence the need for a Step 10.

Validating the curriculum

The draft curriculum has been completed and excitement is running high as the drapes are removed. No one as yet can have any idea as to the effectiveness of the curriculum in meeting the terms of the declared philosophy and model of nursing and the contributory aims, goals and educational objectives which it has been designed to meet. Unfortunately, you cannot run 'sea-trials' with a curriculum on any spare Thursday afternoon, so the only means you have of assessing its validity is to check the whole Curriculum Tabulation (Step 8) most carefully in every respect – in your committee room.

To do this, you should work back from the learning/teaching and assessment techniques, resource provision and proposed subject content, up through the successive stages of educational exercises, requisite knowledge, attitudes and skills, educational objectives which define the requisite changes in the students, the goals, aims, list of tasks and nursing model right up to the nursing philosophy in order to ensure, as far as you can in theory, that provision at each stage of the curriculum fully and appropriately meets the requirements of the next stage above it (see the diagram of this process on page 8).

This means, for example, that the subject content, assuming that it is appropriately taught, resourced and assessed, should, all else being equal, provide appropriate material for the proposed educational exercises and that these, in turn, should produce the changes in the students' knowledge, attitudes and skills that are required by the educational objectives and that the sum of these objectives, in *their* turn, will be sufficiently comprehensive and well-directed as to bring about the goals and aims that will enable students to meet all the nursing 'tasks' in the spirit and the letter of the nursing model and philosophy. Your job in validation is to ensure, on paper at least, that 'all else *is* equal'.

Of course, this can only be an estimate, based upon the draft of your Curriculum Tabulation and a general consensus among all those consulted that this should, in all probability, turn out to be an effective curriculum since everything appears to be in place and appropriate for its function. As regards being 'appropriate for its function', this is a last opportunity to ensure that the curriculum will meet the requirements of the supervisory body. In this country, these are the requirements of the United Kingdom Central Council as expressed in its Training Rules (Nurses, Midwives and Health Visitors Rules Approval Order 1983, No. 873) Appendix B paragraph 18(1). A copy of the relevant paragraph is reproduced as Figure 12.1.

The estimate of validity in no way impinges upon the desirability or relevance of the philosophical aspects of the nursing or educational elements. If there is any residual disagreement about these it can only be dealt with by a complete re-think at the top and a complete re-working of all the aims, goals, objectives and learning/teaching and assessing provisions to match the modified philosophies. At the same time that the theoretical validity of the curriculum is being checked, an attempt should be made to produce a similar estimate of its 'reliability'. This term is used in the rather technical sense of attempting, by consultation with the appropriate authorities, to ascertain the validity of your curriculum when transplanted to other generations of students and to other institutions with different sets of students, teachers, resources and facilities. In theory, it should, if truly valid, be equally reliable in producing consistent and successful results in these new environments, but again this aspect of its potential universality can only be assumed by intuition and discussion of the draft.

Presentation and submission of the curriculum

The presentation of the curriculum will involve a further massive outlay of time, effort and money. By the time the curriculum itself and all the supplementary information about the institution, its policy-making processes and policies, its staff, facilities and existing courses, together with the background details of the proposed curriculum's inception and justification,

United Kingdom Central Council Training Rules APPENDIX B

Nurses, Midwives and Health Visitors Rules
Approval Order 1983 No. 873

18(1)   Courses leading to a qualification the successful completion of which shall enable an application to be made for admission to Part 1 of the register shall provide opportunities to enable the student to accept responsibility for her personal professional development and to acquire the competencies required to:

(a)   Advise on the promotion of health and the prevention of illness
(b)   Recognise situations that may be detrimental to the health and wellbeing of the individual
(c)   Carry out those activities involved when conducting the comprehensive assessment of a person's nursing requirements
(d)   Recognise the significance of the observations made and use these to develop an initial nursing assessment
(e)   Devise a plan of nursing care based on the assessment with the co-operation of the patient, to the extent that this is possible, taking into account the medical prescription
(f)   Implement the planned programme of nursing care and where appropriate teach and co-ordinate other members of the caring team who may be responsible for implementing specific aspects of the nursing care
(g)   Review the effectiveness of the nursing care provided, and where appropriate, initiate any action that may be required
(h)   Work in a team with other nurses, and with medical and para-medical staff and social workers
(i)   Undertake the management of the care of a group of patients over a period of time and organise the appropriate support services

related to the care of the particular type of patient with whom she is likely to come in contact when registered in that Part of the register for which the student intends to qualify.

Examinations

19(1)   To qualify as a person who can apply to be registered in…Part 1…of the register – the student shall:

(c)   Have passed an examination, held or arranged by a Board which may be in parts, and which shall be designed so as to assess the student's theoretical knowledge, practical skills and attitudes and demonstrate her ability to undertake the relevant competencies specified in rule 18 of these rules.

Figure 12.1 United Kingdom Central Council Training Rules.

are committed to typescript, the proposal could well run to over one hundred and fifty pages, with, perhaps, colour-coded chapters and tabulations and smart ring-binders or spiral binding. Consider, too, that every member of the staff and the co-opted members of the curriculum design team should have a personal copy and that copies should be made available to key personnel in the service and management sectors and in the other hospitals and community areas of the Authority.

Presentation is usually made to a supervisory national moderating body whose approval must be sought and obtained for the implementation of the new curriculum and it, too, will need multiple copies. In the case of the English National Board, there are nineteen pages of detailed instructions, with a glossary, for the format, content and timing of 'Applications for approval/reapproval of a course' (Circular 1985/30/MAT). It is reasonable to assume that, since nursing is such a vital element in the national health provision in all countries of the world, and, in most instances, is subject to official government control or oversight, any school or department must expect to be subject to this kind of regulation of its activities in the interests of the maintenance of high standards of service, of education and of the professional integrity of the personnel concerned.

The wider context

A number of important organisational tasks remain to be done before the implementation of the new curriculum. You should:

1. Attempt to identify and deal with elements of the 'hidden' curriculum by either forestalling them or promoting their appearance according to your estimate of the likely value of those which you *are* able to anticipate.
2. Plan the efficient and economical use of all existing resources and ensure that those needed but not immediately available will be made available when required for the implementation of the relevant part of the new curriculum.
3. Advise on the kind of students who may be best fitted to obtain the maximum benefit from the new curriculum if, in fact, any particular characteristics can be shown to be particularly relevant to the demands of the new regime and available among the pool of potential entrants.
4. Advise on the briefing, and, perhaps, re-orientation, of teachers who may have to adapt to the new curriculum in some important professional, practical or personal respects. They will, of course, have been kept in touch with developments and regularly consulted during the process of curriculum design but may not have quite foreseen some of the problems that now appear imminent. This briefing should be one of the last stages in this consultative procedure for the time being.
5. Negotiate the likely date and the timetabling and accommodation for the new curriculum.

Although this agenda may look deceptively brief and innocuous, it does, in fact, involve a great deal of careful thought, planning and delicate negotiation with forces outside the harmonious circle of the curriculum design team. This activity should, perhaps, proceed simultaneously with the printing, binding and presentation of the curriculum and with the lengthy process of obtaining approval for its implementation, otherwise there is little hope of smooth implementation before enthusiasms fade, memories perish and tempers fray. The assumption must therefore be made that the curriculum will be approved in substantially the form in which it was submitted.

Implementation

As regards the actual implementation of the curriculum, following approval by the responsible body, this has already been described in the 'Brief outline' chapter as being rather like delivering up your 'baby' into the hands of others who operate behind closed doors which you are not allowed to open. On second thoughts, at the end of the book and of the process, it may, in more ways than one, be likened to the day when your tempestuous teenager leaves home – to lodge next door!

Chapter 13

Step 10   Reviewing, revising and re-validating the curriculum: evaluation

Reminder

> A cycle of maintaining, modifying and re-validating now takes the place of design and construction activities.

The curriculum design team now has to assume the role of an inspectorate and advisory service in so far as its members are not actively engaged in teaching to the new curriculum. The team may, therefore, decide to change its corporate title to 'Curriculum *Development* Team' at this point. For the foreseeable future members are committed to overseeing the day-by-day progress of learning, teaching and assessing under their curriculum, advising, insisting, trouble-shooting and counselling the casualties. In particular, it is their task to smooth the path of the students who might, quite reasonably, regard themselves as a generation of guinea-pigs. This is a sufficiently onerous burden, but there are graver duties looming ahead.

Neither approval, implementation nor the oversight of learning, teaching and assessing for an unlimited introductory period mark the end of the team's responsibilities for its own creation. Membership of the team may, and probably should, shrink and change as coopted members from other sectors drop out and new blood is introduced to give a fresh and unbiased view of progress and to relieve some of the senior teaching members so that they can return to their normal responsibilities for the direction and administration of the school or department as an institute of learning rather than as a test-bed for a new curriculum.

It has been stressed in the previous Step that the only mode of assessment of the curriculum's performance in relation to its objectives, goals, aims and philosophies has been, at best, the meticulous cross-checking of its provisions, supplemented by informed guess-work on the part of its designers, who can hardly be expected to remain completely impartial in the matter, to establish validity and reliability.

Evaluation

Validation must not be confused with evaluation. This latter activity is only undertaken after the curriculum has been implemented and has been running for some time, say, about a month, at which juncture the opening phase can be examined in the light of evidence accumulated from direct observation of the curriculum *in action* and after the initial period of hourly responses to 'emergencies' has passed. This observation should preferably result in experimental findings made under conditions akin to those required for formal research. This evaluation procedure becomes a routine part of the procedure of curriculum development, as opposed to curriculum design, and usually results in a stream of modifications to the curriculum as weaknesses are revealed under operational pressures and efforts are made to investigate and repair them on a cyclical basis of 'rolling change'.

As opposed to the 'formative' or 'concurrent' estimation of validity which is carried out as the last step in the design process (our Step 9) this is 'summative' evaluation which will last the life of the curriculum – say, about ten years in the normal circumstances of a profession's development and innovation. It ensures, as has been stated, that the validity and reliability of the curriculum are kept under constant surveillance in a self-critical and self-renewing system; that defects are detected and conditions revised and the curriculum re-validated as a whole or in its modified parts until it is working smoothly and producing consistent results of the required standard. It is thereafter reviewed similarly at frequent and regular intervals.

Sources of data for evaluation

One important source of data for evaluation is the student-body, whose assessment results, when analysed in detail, may provide evidence of weaknesses in the system and whose considered opinions elicited by questionnaire or some other form of survey, supplemented by random interviews, may indicate deficiencies which do not show up in assessment results, being, perhaps, of a more administrative or even domestic nature. The students know whether or not they have been changed by their experiences, in what directions and to what extent, even though they may have no clear idea of the significance of the changes in relation to the curriculum objectives.

The teaching staff will also have much to contribute to the process of evaluation since they are probably subject to periodical appraisal in any case and their ability or lack of ability to cope with certain aspects of the curriculum may well be discovered to be due to deficiencies in the curriculum rather than to any deficiencies in their own expertise. They also observe the students daily and assess their work and react to this feedback after they have analysed its roots. However, in a vocational programme, it is important to reach out beyond the narrow confines of the school and to seek a wider evaluation of the students as they carry out work in the wards under the supervision and guidance of clinical teachers or, later, after qualification. Only good can result from involving senior nursing staff from the service sectors in the indirect evaluation of the curriculum by their appraisal of its products, communicated to the curriculum development team in a standardised format for easy analysis. The charges made against the schools of isolation from the mainstream of professional practice would thereby be still further weakened and this evaluation would have the simultaneous effect of creating a useful body of evidence relating to any effort by supervisory or moderating bodies towards the setting of national standards for curriculum-related performance, a tendency which has already begun to invade some sectors of the state education system.

The body of evaluation data focuses upon the clarification of some important educational questions. These include, the overall achievement of students in terms of their pre-course and post-qualification knowledge, attitudes and skills; the making of educational judgements based upon hard evidence as to the overall efficacy of the system; the consideration of internal and external changes in the circumstances that might require modification of the whole curriculum as a matter of necessity or, perhaps, render minor modifications desirable, or marginally advantageous, as the process eventually winds down to the level of 'fine-tuning'; the consideration of the hypothesis, which must be faced – that this might *not* be the best curriculum for the purpose in mind after all; and, in the last event, something not covered by validation, the consideration of any necessary or desirable changes in the philosophies, models, aims and goals themselves which, if approved, would probably lead to the creation, validation and evaluation of a completely new curriculum and course. Evaluation can only proceed by constant experiment and re-thinking of all aspects of the curriculum under review. To most teachers, heavily involved in teaching and absorbed by their task, it understandably remains a major irritant.

Criteria of evaluation studies

The criteria of a successful curriculum evaluation study are relatively few but nevertheless important:

1. It must have *continuity of feedback* from the learners and teachers to the

development team and corresponding continuity in the reactions of the team.

2. There must be an effort to preserve the *delicate structural balance* of such a complex network of integrated elements as a curriculum and any changes proposed in one area must be counterbalanced by tracing the consequences of those changes and making compensatory adjustments there.

3. In view of this degree of integration, every part of the curriculum must be *monitored consistently* to the same high standard of surveillance.

4. It is important that everything is observed with *complete objectivity* and that no corner must be considered sacrosanct and immune to change or rejection. Observations in the affective areas of attitude change must not, however, be given a spurious air of objectivity by wrong-headed attempts to quantify them to an unjustified degree of 'accuracy'.

5. As in the prior process of validation, the question of *validity* arises here but is more complicated than before. 'Content validity' concerns the charting of learning activities at the sharp end of student contact wherever it takes place; 'status validity' describes the extent of the students' formal achievement; 'predictive validity' describes the extent to which such achievement can safely be regarded as an indicator of the students' future behaviour and achievements; 'Construct validity' is the final assurance that all these other measures of validity can be accepted, for evaluation purposes, as accurate and consistent measures of the effect of that part of the curriculum upon students and can be accepted as indicators of the success or failure of the curriculum, rather than of the students, at that point.

Some strategies for evaluation

The responsibility for evaluation rests ultimately with the curriculum development team. Even though evaluation of the work done is a daily function of the teacher, there is a rather natural reluctance to make one's failures, however minor, part of the flow of public knowledge which alone makes evaluation possible. Even discussion with a close colleague will be inhibited if he is a member of, or has indirect contacts with, the curriculum development team.

Informal and impersonal discussion by the team responsible for teaching to the new curriculum can be helpful, especially if there is a substantial representation of the design or development team among the membership, but it may lack precision and academic rigour and rely too much upon impressions of what is going on. Formal discussions by the same team, held at regular intervals as part of the curriculum development routine and using a regular supply of detailed and authentic evidence in acceptable quantitative terms whenever possible, probably constitute the best way to conduct an evaluation process, short of admitting representatives of an external consulting or moderating body, suitably briefed and shorn of their aura of threat to the status quo.

An evaluation study may cover the whole curriculum in one vast operation in order to assess how well it is performing as a whole or it may proceed by examining one element or sector at a time, beginning with those offering immediate and obvious problems or those which are more suspect than others because of known difficulties in the initial process of design and construction. In either case, the procedure must be related to the particular conditions, students, teachers and facilities of a given institution, the vital criterion being, of course, the achievement of the objectives and the furtherance of the philosophy set by the institution in its curriculum as a cornerstone of the work.

Such an evaluation must be carefully planned to look at the right phenomena in the right order and with the right aims in view, pursuing its course with the minimum disruption of whatever is going on, both for the sake of the students who are, after all, studying for a career qualification, and for the sake of the investigators who need to see things as they really are. For these reasons, it may be decided to dispense with the customary pilot study which normally precedes an investigation of this type and degree of rigour. Three methods of proceeding are commonly used in these circumstances:

1. Perhaps the most rigorous method is, in fact, the introduction of the kind of external representatives mentioned above in the form of psychologists who would be particularly skilled in measuring intelligence and attainment and would measure, and produce indices of, the gain in learning achieved by students under the new curriculum over given phases or periods of time. This could, with some difficulty, be applied to the assessment of gains in the adoption of attitudes as well as to gains in the areas of knowledge and skills. The indices of gain are often expressed as a 'paired percentage', for example, '90/90' gain indicates that ninety per cent of the students achieved at least ninety per cent scores on the tests undertaken. These are objective and immediately recognisable and useful measures.

2. A second common strategy used by professional evaluators is often applied in sociological investigations where it is considered difficult or comparatively meaningless or misleading to produce hard statistics. It has been given the name of 'Illuminative evaluation'[1] and is based, not upon quantitative data, but upon a continuous written narrative concerning the curriculum, its context, implementation and developmental trends, moving in close to focus upon areas of special concern. The evaluator shares the life of the population of teachers and students

concerned for the duration of the study, sampling their views, observing their reactions to events, noting the many variables that impinge upon the scene and disqualify any simple conclusions. This evaluator can show not only that a given part of the programme has failed to achieve its objectives, but may also be able to show, if requested to do so, *why* this has happened and what means may be adopted to reverse the failure. Admittedly, there is a substantial element of subjectivity in this type of evaluation, but it is informed, or 'illuminated' evaluation, carried out by an expert who knows what to look for in these 'sociological' situations, maintains detailed and highly relevant notes and eventually carries out a reasonably objective analysis from them and produces a comprehensive, professionally-compiled report that may have a great deal to offer in the way of subtle insights that would be missing from a more rigorously scientific report.

3. A third broad strategy of evaluation employs elements from both of the above methods as and where they may be most helpful, but starts from the point of view of the curriculum design and development teams rather than from that of the 'consumer'. Cognisant of their aims and hopes for the curriculum, the investigator moves into areas which the teams, from their experience, consider to be possible sources or sites of trouble.

Carried out with this degree of determination and rigour, evaluation becomes a permanent and invaluable element in the research and development ethos of the school, providing answers to many questions which might otherwise be dismissed as mere speculation and go unanswered to the detriment of the students and, ultimately, to the detriment of the school and of nursing in general.

References

1. Parlett, Malcolm, Hamilton, David, *Evaluation as illumination: a new approach to the study of innovatory programmes*, Edinburgh, University of Edinburgh Centre for Research in the Educational Sciences, 1972, Occasional paper No. 9. Also described by Parlett in Reason, P.A., Rowan, John (editors), *Human inquiry: a sourcebook of new paradigm research*, Chichester, Wiley, 1981, pp. 219–226.

Further reading

Gallego, Amalia P., *Evaluating the school: a case study in the evaluation of a school of nursing*, London, Royal College of Nursing, 1983, (RCN Research series).

Heath, Jean, *Curriculum design in nursing: a practical guide for course planners*, Sheffield, NHS, (now ENB) Learning Resources Unit, 1982, pp. 52–62.

Further reading

BRITISH BOOKS

Allan, Peta, Jolley, Moya (editors), *The curriculum in nursing education*, London, Croom Helm, 1987.

Allen, Hazel O., Murrell, John (editors), *Nurse training: an enterprise in curriculum development at St. Thomas's Hospital*, Plymouth, Macdonald and Evans, 1978.

Davis, Bryn D. (editor), *Nursing education: research and developments*, London, Croom Helm, 1987 (particularly Chs. 1 and 7).

Department of Education and Science, Further Education Curriculum Review and Development Unit, *Curriculum styles and strategies: a review of styles and strategies of curriculum innovation in secondary (and higher) education and their relevance and applicability to further education*, by Gay Heathcote, Richard Kempa and Iolo Roberts, commissioned from the Department of Education, University of Keele, London, DES, 1983.

Greaves, Fred, *Nurse education and the curriculum: a curricular model*, London, Croom Helm, 1984.

Greaves, Fred, *The nursing curriculum: theory and practice*, London, Croom Helm, 1987.

Heath, Jean, *Curriculum design in nursing: a practical guide for course planners*, Sheffield, NHS (now ENB), Learning Resources Unit, 1982.

Hoy, Ronald A., Moustafa, A.H., Skeath, A., *Balancing the nurse curriculum*, Tunbridge Wells, Costello, 1986.

Stenhouse, Lawrence, *Introduction to curriculum research and development*, London, Heinemann, 1975.

NORTH AMERICAN BOOKS

These appear to be written for academics in the university faculties which are the main seats of nurse education in North America. Nevertheless, some are listed here in the hope that they may provide guidance on some of the theoretical and organisational problems which a practical manual of manageable length must perforce omit or deal with only in passing.

Bevis, Em Olivia, *Curriculum building in nursing: a process*, 3rd edn, St Louis, Missouri, Mosby, 1982.

Pratt, David, *Curriculum design and development*, New York, Harcourt Brace Jovanovich, 1980.

Scales, Freda S., *Nursing curriculum: development, structure, function*, Norwalk, Connecticut, Appleton-Century-Croft, 1985.

Schweer, Jean E. (editor), *Defining behavioral objectives for continuing education offerings in nursing: a four-level taxonomy*, Thorofare, NJ, Slack, 1981.

Torres, Gertrude, Stanton, Marjorie, *Curriculum process in nursing: a guide to curriculum development*, Englewood Cliffs, NJ, Prentice Hall Inc., 1982.

Index